I would like to dedicate this book to my grandmother, Ethel Van Norman, who has always been a special part of my life. At age 83, she has faced many physical and emotional challenges. I admire her determination to meet each challenge head-on and her continued enthusiasm for life and new experiences. I have certainly learned from her that no matter what else occurs in your life you must focus on "enjoying the joy" that is also offered. Grandma, you will never be "old" because your spirit is youthful.

Exercise Programming for Older Adults

Kay A. Van Norman, MS
Montana State University

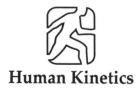

Human Kinetics

Library of Congress Cataloging-in-Publication Data

Van Norman, Kay A., 1957-
    Exercise programming for older adults / Kay A. Van Norman.
      p. cm.
    Includes index.
    ISBN 0-87322-657-7
    1. Exercise for the aged. 2. Physical fitness for the aged.
  I. Title.
GV482.6.V36 1995   94-7497
613.7'044—dc20   CIP

ISBN: 0-87322-657-7

Acquisitions Editor: Rick Frey, PhD
Developmental Editor: Larret Galasyn-Wright
Assistant Editors: Ed Giles and John Wentworth
Copyeditor: Dianna Matlosz
Proofreader: Jim Burns
Indexer: Sheila Ary
Production Manager: Kris Ding
Typesetters and Text Layout: Yvonne Winsor and Ruby Zimmerman
Text Designer: Stuart Cartwright
Cover Designer: Jack Davis
Cover and Interior Photographer: Casey Lipok
Printer: United Graphics

Printed in the United States of America   10 9 8 7 6 5

Human Kinetics
Web site: www.humankinetics.com

United States: Human Kinetics, P.O. Box 5076, Champaign, IL 61825-5076
800-747-4457
e-mail: humank@hkusa.com

Canada: Human Kinetics, 475 Devonshire Road, Unit 100, Windsor, ON N8Y 2L5
800-465-7301 (in Canada only)
e-mail: orders@hkcanada.com

Europe: Human Kinetics, Units C2/C3 Wira Business Park, West Park Ring Road
Leeds LS16 6EB, United Kingdom
+44 (0) 113 278 1708
e-mail: hk@hkeurope.com

Australia: Human Kinetics, 57A Price Avenue, Lower Mitcham, South Australia 5062
08 8277 1555
e-mail: liahka@senet.com.au

New Zealand: Human Kinetics, P.O. Box 105-231, Auckland Central
09-523-3462
e-mail: hkp@ihug.co.nz

Contents

Preface

Exercise Programming for Older Adults is designed to meet the need for a reliable and concise resource on senior exercise. It is written primarily for fitness instructors, health and physical educators, fitness facility managers, and recreation and wellness program directors who want to become knowledgeable about the growing senior exercise market. It will also be a valuable resource for activity directors of senior centers, senior residence facilities, and nursing homes who need information on exercise for older adults. It offers a well-rounded and practical resource that will let readers assess and program for the needs of seniors.

Exercise Programming for Older Adults describes the growth of the senior market and how to reach senior consumers. It also discusses the opportunities this market makes available to fitness and recreation industry managers and instructors. The book provides an overview of the principles of exercise science and a foundation of knowledge on the aging process, the effects of exercise on aging, and the special conditions common in the senior population. It also identifies the special needs of senior exercisers, offers clear guidelines for effectively meeting their needs, and provides specific field-tested land-based and water-based exercises. This well-rounded resource will allow the reader to easily tap into the senior fitness revolution.

Acknowledgments

My first thanks go to my family—to my husband, George Gebhardt, our son, Brock, and our newest arrival, Cole. George, thank you for putting up with my spreading this manuscript out over the kitchen table during the past 2 years, and for your continued support and encouragement throughout the process. Brock, thank you for understanding the many times I said, "Not now. I'm working on the book." Cole, knowing you were coming provided great motivation to finish the manuscript, because I knew that when you arrived I would have very little time for anything extra!

Thanks also go to my mother, Nora Cellers, my sisters, Tommi Hageman and Lori Heaton, and my brother, Jim Van Norman, for believing that I could do this and continuing to expect to see some results. Lori, thanks for all of the phone calls (exactly when I needed them) to help push me through the process of writing—even when I didn't particularly feel like it! Thanks also to my father, Richard Van Norman, who always encouraged me to take on new challenges.

I would like to thank the many people in the Bozeman Young at Heart program. You are the inspiration for this book and my teachers, and you continue to provide me with some wonderful role models for aging.

A special thanks to the models in the book who gave their time so generously: Ruth Seward, Norma Young, Phyllis Craft, Bert and Mo Mokros, Martin Burris, Bill and Mary Walters, Winnie White, and Helen Degidio.

Many thanks to Casey Lipok of Lipok photography in Bozeman, who spent many hours ensuring that the photographs were right and went above and beyond the call of duty to make my job easier. I couldn't have chosen a better photographer.

Special thanks also go to Laurel Dimock and Carol Sanford from the MSU Department of Health and Human Development. You have been great about helping me get the manuscript typed and out the door to meet the always impending deadlines.

Last, I'd like to add a note of appreciation to the people in the Council on Aging and Adult Development. I appreciate their dedication to providing quality exercise programming for seniors and their willingness to share knowledge and provide encouragement.

CHAPTER 1

Aging and Fitness

Exercise programs meeting the special needs of the senior population will soon be in tremendous demand. How am I so sure? There are several reasons. First, the percentage of the population aged 55 and over is steadily and dramatically increasing. More and more information is available on the health benefits of regular exercise for seniors, and the public is becoming aware of the role exercise plays in maintaining a positive quality of life well into advanced age.

We are finding out that many seniors can remain physically active, and our expectations of what the "golden years" should be like are changing. Seniors need no longer resign themselves to a life-style of inactivity and deteriorating health. Older adults are realizing that they can take an active role in maintaining and improving their health through regular exercise, and they will demand exercise classes that safely meet their special needs.

We can expect this demand to make a significant impact on the fitness industry and to open many avenues of career growth for fitness professionals. The field of senior fitness, currently small, will be one of the fastest growing markets in the fitness industry—and perhaps one of its largest.

AGING WORLD POPULATIONS

The past few years have seen a considerable increase in the number of research papers, magazine and journal articles, and books devoted to the "graying of America." According to census data presented in "Aging America: Trends and Projections" (U.S. Senate, 1988), in 1900 fewer than 1 in 10 Americans was 55 or older, and 1 in 25 was 65 or older. By 1989 the proportions had risen to 1 in 5 Americans at least 55 years old and 1 in 8 at least 65. Projections show a continual uphill climb— more than 1 in 5 Americans are expected to be 65 or older by the year 2030. America is not alone in this phenomenon. Many European countries, Japan, and Canada are also projecting large increases in their senior populations. Figure 1.1 illustrates the projected aging of the populations of several developed countries. Note the especially large increases expected in Canada and Japan, where the numbers of people 65+ will nearly double. Over the next 30 years the relatively youthful Japan will catch up to and exceed the rest of the developed world in regard to the proportion of its population aged 65+. A further review of the literature indicates that many developed countries are struggling with similar issues and problems presented by a shift from a youthful population toward one dominated by older adults.

UNITED STATES

In the United States analysts from many disciplines are focusing on the scope of problems posed by the dramatic increase of older adults. Of major concern is the effect these increases will have on a health care industry already in crisis, plagued by spiraling costs and an increasing shortage of professionals. An aging America will mean a proportional increase in many long-term health problems, a potentially crushing burden. It also poses some interesting challenges to the "sandwich generation," who will be under tremendous economic strain to provide care for dependent children at the

same time they are trying to provide care for aging parents (Ostroff, 1989).

According to "Aging America: Trends and Projections" (U.S. Senate, 1988), from the year 2005 to 2025 the aging of the baby boomers will create the fastest rate of growth in the American older adult population. The 65 to 79 age group will grow 10 times faster during this era than it has for the past 15 years. It is important to note that the baby boomers as a group have routinely had a significant impact on public policy. Some analysts warn that the expected growth in social programs to address the needs and wants of the senior population will occur at the expense of those in the diminishing work force (primarily made up of the already financially burdened "sandwich generation"). Providing more programs for the aged may also have a negative impact on those social and health programs, already seriously underfunded, aimed at American youth. Amidst all of these concerns and conflicts American marketing firms are rushing to develop strategies for capitalizing on the needs and wants of the emerging senior population (Thompson, 1990).

JAPAN

As Japan's aged population spirals upward it is also struggling with significant social issues. Dentzer (1991) points out that health and pension costs will increase at the same time that Japan faces severe labor shortages. The "national burden," defined as the sum of all taxes plus all other payments workers make to fund Japan's universal health insurance and pension systems, is projected to rise from the current 41% to just under 50% by the year 2020.

In addition, the health care system for Japanese elderly is already experiencing serious problems. According to Dentzer, there now is a wait of up to 2 years for admission to Tokyo nursing homes. In turn, this wait lengthens the average hospital stay for a person over age 70 to 95 days (compare this with an average stay of 8.5 days for people over 70 in the U.S.). On the business and industry side of the issue lies a hint of international conflict. As in the automotive industry, the Japanese health services industry strives to prevent non-Japanese firms from providing major services and products for the Japanese elderly (Dentzer, 1991).

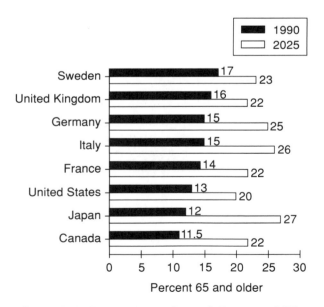

Figure 1.1 Percentages of populations aged 65 and older in selected countries in 1990 and projected for 2025. Note: Data from U.S. Bureau of the Census, International Data Base.

EUROPE

European countries also face many severe problems arising from the changing structure of the work force and the need for socioeconomic provisions for an aging population. The emerging imbalances between age groups create potentially negative impacts on living conditions, patterns of consumption, and government-supported medical and health care provisions for the aged. The cost of generous services for the elderly in Norway and Sweden, for example, have helped push their national burden to approximately 60% (Dentzer, 1991). In addition, Europe's large aging population and their increasing demands for products and services will undoubtedly have a significant impact on the changing European economic structure.

EXERCISE AND HEALTH IN AN AGING AMERICA

Clearly, efforts must begin now to prepare for and where possible to control what could be the devastating effects of an aging world population. The problems common to most countries with aging populations stem from conditions normally associated with advanced age: the loss of health (i.e., a strain on health care systems); the loss of productivity (i.e., a diminished work force); and the loss of independence (i.e., a need for long-term care provisions for the aged) (U.S. Senate, 1988). As government and business interests search for ways to contain the enormous medical costs associated with an aging population, both entities will enthusiastically support the move toward healthy life-styles as preventive medicine. In much the same way that the auto insurance industry now offers safe driver incentives, the health insurance industry is looking toward offering incentives for healthy life-styles. In the past decade there has been a flood of research focusing on the positive effect exercise has on improving and maintaining health. This research consistently supports the theory that disuse is a significant factor in the loss of function and the diminished level of health formerly accepted as normal aging (Office of Disease Prevention and Health Promotion, 1990). Therefore, involvement in regular exercise will undoubtedly

be one of the key elements identified in a healthy life-style. The new "age-sensitive" media is also likely to focus increasing amounts of attention on the volume of research documenting the importance of exercise in retarding the physical decline associated with aging. By enabling older adults to maintain good health, exercise can play a significant role in slowing the growth of the health care crises, the diminished levels of productivity, and the rise in dependent care.

MAINTAINING HEALTHSPAN

Recently in *Healthy People 2000* (ODPHP, 1990), the United States Department of Health and Human Services offered public testimony that a sedentary life-style is a leading factor in premature disability and death in the United States. They went on to strongly state that regular exercise is a critical aspect of a healthy life-style. It is clear that whereas improved health care helps increase lifespan, regular exercise helps increase "healthspan," the length of time that a person can enjoy a healthy, active, positive quality of life. Improving the healthspan of older adults could dramatically lessen the impact of an aging population on the health care industry.

MAINTAINING PRODUCTIVITY

Maintaining good health also lengthens the amount of time that a person can remain a productive part of society. Currently analysts on aging issues are noting that retirement-age adults who are in good health are showing a preference toward remaining in the work force. The predictions are that many seniors will retire from one profession only to begin another. This factor will have a positive effect on the problem of a diminishing work force.

MAINTAINING INDEPENDENCE

The contribution regular exercise makes toward healthspan will significantly increase the amount of time that a senior can maintain an independent life-style. According to "Aging America: Trends and Projections" (U.S. Senate, 1988), 8 million of the current 30 million adults 65 or over live alone. When older adults live alone it is critical that they be able to take care of their most basic personal needs. To be considered independent, a person must be able to bathe, dress, transfer (get in and out of beds and chairs), walk, eat, and go to the toilet without assistance (Rogers, Rogers, & Branch, 1989). Loss of any of these functions requires dependence on some form of long-term care. The fastest growing segment of the population is the 85+ group with a reported 56% of adults over 75 restricted to some degree in daily activities. Therefore, senior exercise programs that focus on maintaining functional fitness (i.e., the level of fitness necessary for an individual to take care of personal needs and maintain an independent life-style) will undoubtedly play a large role in curbing the increasing need for long-term care provisions for the elderly.

NEW ATTITUDES TOWARD AGING

The aging baby boomer generation appears to have vastly different expectations of what their advanced years can and should be like. According to Ostroff (1989), the baby boomers have forged an identity as the youth generation and with the enthusiastic support of business and media have focused their attention on youth and all of its advantages. As the youth generation, baby boomers are unwilling to accept the image of advanced age coupled with a sedentary life-style, declining physical health, and senility. Instead, with their considerable economic clout they are changing public opinion concerning older adults. The media who less than 5 years ago consistently portrayed seniors as "sweet little old ladies" or "doddering old fools" has received the message and dramatically changed its approach to avoid offending this large block of consumers (Thompson, 1990). Youth-oriented baby boomers are also unwilling to accept without question a significant decline in their functional ability and quality of life simply due to age, and appear willing to take every measure feasible to counteract or slow the aging process. Marketing specialists speculate that in this quest for the "fountain of youth" baby boomers will create

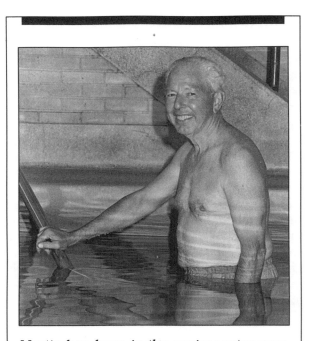

Martin has been in the senior water aerobics class for 9 years, and his lean, muscular body shows the obvious effects of an active lifestyle. He would easily be able to attend an exercise class with people much younger—so, why does he prefer the senior exercise class? Martin says he is very comfortable with the exercises offered in the classes for seniors because they help him maintain ease of movement without aggravating the arthritis he has throughout his body. If he misses a week or two of class, Martin says, he notices a definite pain and stiffness in his muscles and joints. "Music that I enjoy listening to and an instructor who has enthusiasm for teaching are also important to me," he says. Martin also mentions that he likes exercising with the other seniors at the 8 a.m. class. "Our group of early birds has been exercising together for the past 9 years. It's a great way to start the day with people that you have come to know and enjoy."

a tremendous demand for what the health and fitness industry has to offer, including athletic equipment, exercise and fitness centers, weight reduction centers, rehabilitation services, wellness-oriented publications, and fitness vacations or camps (Ostroff, 1989).

CHANGING FITNESS NEEDS

Fitness continues to be a significant component in the quest to maintain youth. Of great importance, however, is that along with the changing attitudes about aging will come the necessary changing fitness needs of this group. The focus will shift away from the ideal of a "hard-body" or super athletic fitness toward the concept of fitness that maintains and improves the quality of everyday life. The baby boomer generation has had a significant impact on our society, collectively demanding that their needs and wants be met by business, industry, and social services (Cutler, 1989), and as their exercise needs change, they will also demand that this important need be adequately met.

Older adult exercisers will be looking for safe, low-impact exercise programs that enhance overall fitness, including cardiovascular endurance, strength, flexibility, coordination, and balance. However, because an older adult population has a significantly higher risk of arthritis, osteoporosis, diabetes, joint and muscular dysfunction, and cardiovascular dysfunction (conditions that significantly affect exercise safety), senior exercisers will require programming that addresses these risks. The challenge to the fitness industry will be to provide senior exercise programs that address the elements of fitness while balancing the benefits with the risks the activity could pose to older participants. While striving to meet this challenge the fitness industry will encounter a wide range of functional ability among senior consumers. The older fitness consumer will be made up of three main groups, each requiring significant differences in programming. However, the exercise needs for each will remain centered around a safe, effective, senior-sensitive approach to fitness.

HEALTHY FIT SENIORS

The first group will be those who have been committed to exercise throughout young adulthood and will continue through advanced age. Many of these seniors will be high functioning and may be able to successfully attend an average exercise class at a fitness facility, or may be self-motivated enough to pursue a personal fitness routine. Many others will welcome a seniors' class that provides them with an opportunity to exercise without feeling that they have to compete with students who are 20 years younger, more vigorous, and easily able to perform the exercises. In addition they will enjoy being with people of their own age and interests and exercising with music that suits their tastes.

HEALTHY UNFIT SENIORS

Another group of seniors will be those who have exercised sporadically throughout young adulthood. Although they know it is good for them, they have never really committed to a regular schedule of exercise. At some point these seniors will notice a significant decline in physical capacity. Without regular exercise the average person will begin gradually losing physical function in the early 30s. The level of functioning will markedly decline by the time such people reach their early 60s (Elkowitz & Elkowitz, 1986).

Many seniors in this category will make a commitment to exercise when they experience this diminished level of function. These seniors will not be able to successfully attend an average exercise class at a fitness facility. Many will fail to keep up, leaving class feeling "It's too late, I may as well accept that I am getting old." Others, trying to keep up, will likely suffer a series of injuries that will eventually make it impossible for them to continue. These seniors must have access to an exercise program that takes into account their decline in physical function without treating them as if they are incapable of performing exercise that will increase their present level of function. By attending an exercise class specifically designed for seniors, they will successfully complete the majority of movements while being at minimal risk for injury. By observing others their age and older successfully and vigorously exercising, they will be encouraged and excited about their newly made commitment to fitness.

PHYSICALLY RESTRICTED SENIORS

This group includes those who have experienced some type of illness or injury that has significantly diminished their physical function, such as cardiovascular disease, diabetes, arthritis, osteoporosis, and muscle and joint dysfunction. Exercise may be the medically prescribed course of action for rehabilitation from injury or to slow the progression of symptoms of the illness. These seniors have absolutely no chance of benefiting from a typical exercise class at a fitness facility. They will require a safe, effective seniors' class carefully designed to provide them with a beneficial amount of exercise without putting them at risk of further dehabilitation.

The Fitness Industry And An Aging Population

Our aging society, the new focus on exercise as preventive medicine, altered expectations of advanced age, and the changing exercise needs of older adults are all factors indicating that there will be tremendous growth in the senior exercise market. The fitness industry can utilize many of the strategies developed by the general business world to effectively analyze the needs of their older fitness consumers. Of special concern to the fitness industry are the obvious changes occurring in their "average" fitness consumer, and the identified mature-market niches of health care, leisure time, and products that combat aging. In addition close attention should be given to strategies for effectively using the media to reach the older adult consumer. The demand created for fitness classes and other health-related activities that meet the special needs of older adults will make a large impact on the fitness industry by providing a wide range of opportunities for fitness facilities and professionals.

Fitness Facilities: A New Market

The fitness industry is already seeing a growth in the older adult market. As a result, fitness facilities are in a transition from their primary focus on the young adult market to other areas

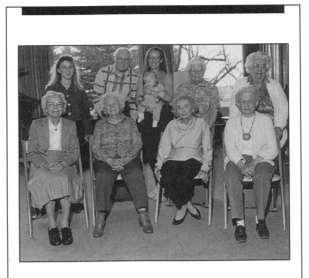

A discussion of the advantages of the senior exercise market for fitness instructors could not be complete without speaking to the many personal rewards of working with older adults. It is a pleasure to work with people who are enthusiastic about what exercise does for them and who are committed to improving the quality of their lives. I also enjoy the personal relationships that are open for development inside and outside of class time. My senior students like to hear about what is happening in my life and with my young family. It is fun to share this information and then gain insights from them on how life patterns change as families grow. As a young adult with what sometimes seem like overwhelming job and family responsibilities, I am grateful that through listening to the thoughts of older adults I am better able to keep my own life in balance. I credit my relationship with senior students for the development of what I call my "perspective check." When a situation arises that begins to create stress, I find myself asking, Will it matter tomorrow? Next week? Next year? In 5 years? If I can answer these questions all yes, then the situation may be worth some anxiety. But I seldom get past the next-week question before I answer no, and with that I can immediately put the problem into its proper perspective.

such as corporate, families, and the older adult markets. Focusing on the older adult market will necessitate a change in emphasis from "superfitness" toward fitness as stress reduction and the key to improving general health. There will be an increase in classes such as low-impact aerobics, walking programs, and water aerobics that better meet the needs of older adults who seek aerobic conditioning. There will also be an increase in classes such as light weight lifting, t'ai chi, circuit training, and chair exercise, which help maintain functional fitness by focusing on improvement of strength, range of motion, coordination, and balance. Providing a range of classes that meet the needs of a variety of levels of functional ability will ensure an increase in the senior exercise market by dramatically increasing the number of consumers to whom fitness facilities can provide a valuable service. An additional advantage of the senior market is that it allows for a significant increase in the number of exercisers a facility can serve without overcrowding during the traditional peak hours of 6 to 8 a.m., noon, and 5 to 7 p.m. (corresponding to the 8 to 5 workday). With many seniors retired or in a flexible job situation, senior exercise classes can be scheduled to utilize nonpeak hours. Increased clientele and better utilization of the fitness facility are obvious incentives, and fitness facility managers will aggressively pursue the senior consumer.

FITNESS INSTRUCTORS: CHALLENGES AND OPPORTUNITIES

The rise of the senior fitness market will also provide challenges and opportunities for fitness instructors. The challenges will be to become educated in the special needs of the senior exerciser and knowledgeable on how to safely meet these needs. Instructors will need specific strategies for managing the higher risks associated with programming for an older adult population that exhibits a high incidence of diminished vision and hearing and may suffer to varying degrees from debilitating illnesses. In addition, many older adults will exhibit significant muscle weakness, compromising their ability to safely participate in vigorous movement. Instructors will need to understand how the motivations of the average senior exerciser (to maintain functional fitness and a positive quality of life) differ from those of the young adult population. In addition, the social and emotional components will become an increasingly important part of exercise programming, making it necessary for the fitness instructor to plan ways to facilitate their development within the structure of the class.

Fitness instructors who understand and effectively administer to the needs of the older fitness consumer will be in high demand in the fitness industry. In addition to increased teaching opportunities there will also be unlimited opportunities for the fitness professional who wishes to branch out into some of the mature-market niches associated with healthy life-styles. For example, Ostroff (1989) speculates that the travel and leisure industry will experience significant growth as a result of the aging of America. He further speculates that a hot spot for growth in the travel industry will be the creation of health and fitness-oriented vacation packages that cater to the active older adult. Part of this package will be a qualified senior exercise specialist. There will also be vast opportunities in the area of products and services that help the senior consumer counter the effects of aging. Personal fitness trainers who specialize in older adult fitness and fitness products designed specifically to assist the older adult will be in demand. There will also be a demand for fitness professionals who can educate others on the special needs of senior exercisers and how to safely and effectively meet these needs. Clearly, the rapidly growing senior exercise market is wide open for any who wish to take a leadership role. As a fitness professional the opportunities to make a difference in the senior exercise field are numerous. There is also the rewarding knowledge that this specialized field makes a significant contribution to improving quality of life for others.

CHAPTER 2

Exercise Science and Age-Related Changes in Functional Ability

To work safely and effectively with older adults you must understand the basic principles of exercise science. This understanding should include the basic principles of exercise physiology and how they apply to exercise training, the functional systems of the body and how they interact, and the basic musculoskeletal structure and how it interacts with the body's other systems to create movement. It is a true advantage to have background in health or physical education providing some depth of knowledge in the area of exercise science. Although there is no substitute for a thorough understanding, you can acquire the basic understanding necessary to develop a good exercise program. If you do not have formal education in exercise science, take the time to study the resources available in this area. *The Aerobic Dance-Exercise Instructor Manual*, chapters 1 (by Christine Wells) and 2 (by Ellen

Kreighbaum), provides a clear, concise picture of the elements of physiology and of anatomy and kinesiology. Locate a good visual chart that identifies the bones of the skeleton and all of the major muscle groups for easy and frequent reference. Look for anatomy and biomechanics lab manuals designed for college classes. Many catalogs that offer fitness products also provide skeleton and muscle diagrams. The diagrams describing which muscles are responsible for creating specific movements are very helpful. Talk to a physical education professional, a physical therapist, or some other health professional who deals with the movement of the body. Study your resources, and then ask these movement professionals specific questions to determine if your understanding is correct.

You also must understand the normal aging process and the positive effect exercise has on slowing this process. Normal aging is characterized by a gradual decline of function in the various systems of the body, excluding those losses that are the result of disease or injury. The positive effect exercise has on slowing this functional decline has been well documented (MacRae, 1986; Stamford, 1988; Smith & Gilligan, 1989). Finally you must have a basic knowledge of the special conditions likely to occur in an older adult population and how they affect exercise potential and safety.

The information in this manual is simply a brief overview of the foundation knowledge necessary to provide quality programming for seniors and gives you a starting point for further investigation. Do not be intimidated about seeking a further understanding in these important areas. Aggressively expanding your knowledge base will help you assure that the exercises you offer your senior participants are both safe and effective.

EXERCISE PHYSIOLOGY AND AGING SYSTEMS

Exercise physiology is the study of how the body functions during exercise. It provides the basis for understanding how the body functions at rest and how these functions change during exercise. It also provides an understanding of how the body adapts to exercise training (Wells, 1987). Exercise physiology examines these functions at the cellular level providing an understanding of the different metabolic systems. An important principle for the fitness instructor to understand is the principle of specificity. Very generally, this principle of training states that physiological adaptations (i.e., changes brought about by exercise) are specific to the system(s) that are overloaded or stressed with exercise. For example, aerobic metabolism requires a constant supply of oxygen, so aerobic exercise must consist of the types of movement that can be performed continuously over a relatively long period of time without creating oxygen deprivation. Anaerobic metabolism, on the other hand, does not require a replenishment of oxygen and is characterized by quick, explosive movements that can only be performed for relatively short periods of time. Using running as

an example, the principle of specificity dictates that if you wish to develop cardiorespiratory endurance, you must provide movements that maintain a constant supply of oxygen, such as jogging, thus allowing aerobic metabolism. If you wish to develop the ability to perform fast, explosive actions, you must provide movement that requires anaerobic metabolism, such as sprinting. Exercise programming for seniors, which focuses on maintaining the level of physical fitness necessary to enjoy a positive quality of life (i.e., functional fitness), does not use movements that call for anaerobic metabolism.

Another example of specificity would be that to improve muscle strength in the upper body, you must exercise those muscles against resistance (such as weight lifting). Low-impact aerobics or other exercises that utilize the upper body during exercise may show some minimal improvements in muscle endurance but to achieve significant gains in strength, the muscles of the upper body must be overloaded or stressed with exercise. When programming exercise for seniors, it is important to note that weight lifting should be limited to low to moderate weights or low- to medium-resistance stretch bands that allow for 8 to 12 repetitions of each exercise.

CARDIOPULMONARY SYSTEM

The cardiovascular system, composed of the heart and the blood vessels, circulates blood throughout the body. The heart is a muscle that becomes stronger through regular aerobic exercise. A stronger heart muscle is a more efficient pump requiring less frequent contractions to circulate the amount of blood the body requires to function. Aerobic exercise also benefits the blood vessels by helping them maintain their essential elasticity and increasing the number of capillaries. The capillaries take the blood, supplied by the heart and delivered by the blood vessels, and distribute it to the tissues (Kreighbaum, 1987).

The pulmonary system consists of the lungs and the respiratory tract. The lungs receive blood from the heart and fill the blood with oxygen (inhaled air). Then the carbon dioxide (exhaled air) is carried off and expelled through the respiratory tract. The work that the cardiovascular system and the pulmonary system do together to provide oxygen to the rest of the body is called the cardiopulmonary or cardio-respiratory function.

Effects of Aging

The aging of the cardiopulmonary system is associated with a number of important factors. One is the diminished level of oxygen transfer related to respiratory function, cited by MacRae (1986) as being the result of a loss of elasticity of the lung tissue, rigidity of the chest wall, and decreased strength in the respiratory muscles. This combination of conditions contributes significantly to a decrease in cardio-pulmonary endurance. Other factors are a decrease in both stroke volume (the volume of blood pumped from the heart during one heartbeat) and maximum heart rate (the highest heart rate a person can attain). The decline in maximum heart rate is estimated to be approximately 6.3% per decade of age resulting in an estimated maximum heart rate of 195 beats per minute for a 25-year-old, compared to a maximum heart rate of 170 beats per minute for a 65-year-old (Shephard, 1989). Decreases in stroke volume and maximum heart rate both contribute to diminished cardiac output (the amount of blood pumped by the heart per minute). Finally, there are increases in blood pressure (the pressure exerted by the blood on the walls of the arteries) and other vessel-related difficulties (MacRae, 1986). All of these factors contribute significantly to the decline of performance in cardiopulmonary endurance activities that is associated with aging. An aging cardiopulmonary system also demonstrates increased levels of blood lipids, a decreased glucose tolerance, and a decreased sensitivity to insulin. These changes can result in an increased risk of atherosclerosis and adult onset diabetes (MacRae, 1986).

Benefits of Exercise

Regular aerobic exercise has been documented to have a significant positive effect on the car-diopulmonary system thus slowing and even reversing the decline in efficiency associated with the aging of this sytem (MacRae, 1986; Shephard, 1989; Stamford, 1988). Aerobic exercise is credited with increasing respiratory function, maintaining the stroke volume, and reducing resting blood pressure in both younger and older participants. In addition, exercise reduces the level of blood lipids and increases glucose tolerance and insulin sensitivity thus reducing the risk of atherosclerosis and adult onset diabetes (MacRae, 1986). Studies also indicate that there is a greater decline in the efficiency of oxygen transfer in sedentary individuals than in those who are physically active. It is clearly documented that exercise has a significant impact on reducing the loss of aerobic power and endurance associated with aging. It is encouraging to note that the cardiopulmonary system responds to training regardless of previous physical activity patterns (Stamford, 1988).

THE NERVOUS SYSTEM

The nervous system acts as the "computer" controlling all of the bodily functions. The nervous system consists of the central nervous system (the brain and spinal cord) and the peripheral nervous system (pairs of nerve branches originating from the central nervous system). As the nerves branch out, they continue to subdivide until they integrate with the muscle. The last nerve fiber has branches that attach to the skeletal muscle fibers and stimulate the muscle to contract (Kreighbaum, 1987).

Effects of Aging

The nervous system sends and receives all messages processed by the body and is responsible for the actions resulting from these messages. As the nervous system ages the ability to receive, process, and transmit messages slows, resulting in a slower reaction to these messages. In the aging nervous system, there also seems to be an increased reliance on reactive control (using feedback to initiate corrective movement) rather than predictive control (initiating movement in anticipation of a change). Whereas a younger person has the ability to use either control function on demand, an older individual may gradually lose the option of predictive control, necessarily relying then only on reactive control. The decline in reaction and movement times and the use of reactive, rather than predictive, control contributes to the documented decline in efficiently performing tasks requiring speed (Stelmach & Goggin, 1989).

The reduced speed of response holds considerable practical importance, because rapid responses are needed to adequately function in many daily living tasks, such as operating motor vehicles and preventing falls (MacRae, 1989). In addition there is a decline in sensory perception, such as vision and hearing, that may stem from the decreased level of glucose utilization in the brain structures associated with vision, audition, and sensorimotor function (MacRae, 1986). Declines in reaction time, movement time, predictive control, and sensory perception appear to be responsible for the decline of coordination, balance, and agility associated with aging.

Benefits of Exercise

Through regular exercise the slowing of reaction and movement time can be minimized. Studies by Stelmach and Goggin (1989) and Smith and Gilligan (1989) demonstrate that physically trained seniors have much faster reaction times than untrained seniors and that faster reaction times can be gained through practice. Additional studies cited by MacRae (1989) indicate an increase in regional cerebral blood flow in response to exercise that can affect areas of the brain associated with motor function. MacRae also reports that aerobic exercise training in previously sedentary older adults can improve many neuropsychological functions, such as response time, visual organization, memory, and mental flexibility. As stated by MacRae and evidenced by research, "Physical activity may be one of the most powerful interventions currently available for combating the deterioration in functional capacity that occurs with the aging of the central nervous system" (1989, p. 75).

THE MUSCULOSKELETAL SYSTEM

The skeletal system consists of the bones, their articulations (joints), and the tendons and ligaments that hold each articulation together. All movements of the skeletal system take place at the articulations. The muscular system consists of the muscles and their tendinous attachments and provides the forces that cause the bones to move. Each muscle is attached to at least two bones and crosses one or more joints (Kreighbaum, 1987). The interaction of the skeletal system and the muscular system creates a musculoskeletal lever system, which allows movement to occur.

If you visualize the skeleton as a puppet with the muscles as the strings it will help you understand how this lever system creates movement. Consider how a puppet string can only *pull* the puppet parts through a movement (such as pulling an arm up until it is parallel with the floor) or control the effects of gravity on a part (such as slowly lowering the raised arm to the side instead of allowing it to drop forcefully). Clearly, a string cannot push a puppet part through movement. Like the strings on a puppet, the muscles cannot push the skeleton through movement. Muscles can do only one of two things: (a) shorten or contract to pull the bone through movement (concentric contraction) or (b) attempt to shorten in response to some other resistive force, such as gravity. In the latter case, their attempt to shorten is thwarted by the larger force and thus the muscle is pulled or stretched out, lengthening against the resistance (eccentric contraction).

A working knowledge of this system is essential to understanding which muscles are responsible for the movements of each body part. This knowledge will allow you to create an exercise program using "movement that matters" for seniors. For example, the quadriceps muscle helps seniors get up from and down onto chairs, to walk, and to climb stairs. To exercise the quadriceps muscle you must know that it is responsible for extension (increasing the angle) of the knee joint. Therefore exercises that extend (straighten) the knee joint will utilize the quadriceps muscle. Creating additional resistance against extension, such as adding a weight to the ankle, will make the quadriceps muscle work harder to extend the knee, thus contributing to improved strength. Similarly, the hamstring muscle is responsible for flexion (decreasing the angle) of the knee joint. Therefore exercises that flex (bend) the knee joint will utilize the hamstring muscle.

Creating additional resistance (such as adding an ankle weight) will make the hamstring muscle work harder to flex the knee, thus contributing to improved strength. However, when considering adding weight to an exercise, remember to balance the benefits with the risks by taking into account the many special conditions that occur in the senior population.

Effects of Aging

The aging of the musculoskeletal system is related to a number of factors. Diminished muscular strength and endurance of the muscles is partially attributed to a decrease in the number and size of muscle fibers present in the older adult (Buskirk & Segal, 1989). There is additional evidence that with age the muscle fibers respond more slowly to nerve stimulation and with a less efficient muscle reflex (Anspaugh, Ezell, Rienzo, Varnes, & Walker, 1989). The loss of muscle mass and responsiveness results in an estimated loss in strength of 25–30% by age 70 (Elkowitz & Elkowitz, 1986). Severe loss of muscle mass resulting in ankle weakness is responsible for many of the falls suffered by adults of advanced age (see Figure 2.1).

Another characteristic of the aging musculoskeletal system is the general loss of muscle mass, which contributes to the overall decline in lean body mass (the mass of the body—muscles, bones, nerves, skin, and organs—excluding the fatty tissue). Some researchers believe that the loss of lean body mass strongly contributes to the decline in basal metabolic rate (the minimum energy required to maintain life processes in a resting state) which in turn contributes to the increase in stored body fat (Stamford, 1988). Muscle flexibility also demonstrates a marked decline. This decline is due to a decrease in muscle fiber flexibility and to decreased elasticity of connective tissue (Stamford, 1988). In addition there is a decline in joint flexibility and stability relating to changes in the joint components of cartilage, ligaments, and tendons (MacRae, 1986). The overall loss of flexibility due to aging of the muscles and joints is estimated at 25% to 30% by age 70 (Elkowitz & Elkowitz, 1986).

The final factor associated with the aging of the musculoskeletal system is the decline of the structural integrity of this system, most significantly affected by a decline in bone mass and bone mineral content. Bone loss in females is reported to begin around age 35 with a resultant 30% loss by approximately age 70. In males, bone loss usually begins at around 50 years of age and results in a 15–20% loss by age 70 (Elkowitz & Elkowitz, 1986; Stamford, 1988). This high rate of bone loss, especially in women, contributes to the higher rate of bone fractures experienced by older adults compared to younger adults.

Benefits of Exercise

Extensive research documents exercise-induced improvements in the musculoskeletal system (MacRae, 1986). These improvements include increases in muscular strength, muscular endurance, lean body mass, joint flexibility, and bone mineral content.

Muscular strength and endurance can be increased in the elderly through training. It is interesting to note that the hypertrophy (increase in muscle size) normally observed in the trained muscle mass of a young individual is not as exaggerated as that of an older individual. Therefore, improved strength in the older individual may be largely due to the increased ability to recruit motor units (a motor neuron

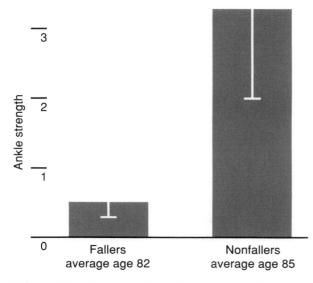

Figure 2.1　Older adults with strong ankles are less likely to fall.
From *Physical Frailty: A Reducible Barrier to Independence for Older Americans* (1990), National Institute on Aging.

and all of the muscle fibers it activates) observed in the trained muscle of an older adult (Stamford, 1988). As expected, the greatest increases in muscular strength and muscular endurance occur when both weight training *and* aerobic training programs are used (MacRae, 1986).

Exercise also significantly slows the loss of lean body mass by helping to prevent and restore the loss of muscle mass (MacRae, 1986; Smith & Gilligan, 1989). In addition regular exercise can reduce fat accumulation, which is closely linked with loss of lean body mass and the resultant decline in basal metabolic rate. Stamford (1988) indicates that older persons can demonstrate a level of body fatness similar to that of younger people if they have a consistent physically active history throughout life. Stamford also suggests that exercise, even when initiated late in life, can still bring about a modest positive change in body composition.

Research also documents the improvement of muscle flexibility in older individuals with exercise (Smith & Gilligan, 1989). One of the studies they examined recorded the same amount of improvement in flexibility between a young group (ages 15–19) and an older group (ages 63–88) who each participated in a 6-week training program. MacRae (1986) reports that improvements in flexibility have also been noted in participants who were involved in a nonstrenuous progressive program as well as in those involved in a more strenuous jogging and cycling program.

Evidence suggests that inactivity and the resultant lack of mechanical force applied to bones is a key factor in bone changes and bone loss (Stamford, 1988). When bone loss declines to such a level that fractures occur with minimal trauma, the integrity of the musculoskeletal system is severely diminished. This weakened state of bone is called osteoporosis and is responsible for a high percentage of fractures in older women (MacRae, 1986). MacRae indicates that improvements in bone mineral content in older adults with severe bone loss is possible with a 3-day-a-week moderate exercise program. Exercise training, through its prevention of bone loss and its contribution to increases in bone mineral content, is a definite factor in retardation of osteoporosis.

It is obvious from the literature that exercise plays a significant role in diminishing the effects of aging on the musculoskeletal system. Exercise is a significant factor in helping prevent the physical frailty that eventually results in complete functional impairment (see Figure 2.2).

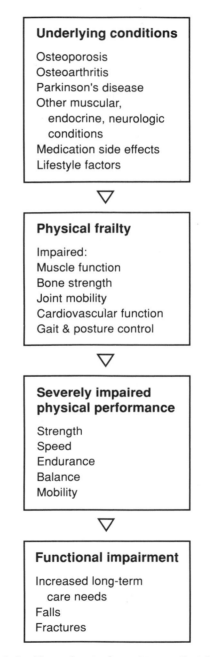

Figure 2.2   Flow chart of conditions that lead to impairment but which can be offset by regular exercise. From *Physical Frailty: A Reducible Barrier to Independence for Older Americans* (1990), National Institute on Aging.

PHYSICAL CONDITIONS REQUIRING SPECIAL CONSIDERATION

Several health conditions occurring at a high rate in the older adult population require special considerations when programming exercise for seniors. Because they affect exercise potential and safety, specific exercise modifications may be required to ensure safe participation. I will discuss only the conditions most frequently encountered and those that can most significantly compromise the safety of your exercise program.

HYPERTENSION (HIGH BLOOD PRESSURE)

Hypertension is the most prevalent disease in adults aged 65 and over. It afflicts close to 1/3 of Americans over the age of 65 and is a primary risk factor in heart disease, coronary artery disease, and affliction by a stroke (American College of Sports Medicine, 1991b; Goldberg & Hagberg, 1990). Those with hypertension are reported to be at risk for a stroke at a level three times higher than nonhypertensives, and at risk for congestive heart failure at a level two times higher than nonhypertensives (Hagberg, 1988). An ACSM study (1991a) identifies two types of hypertension—primary (whose cause is unknown) and secondary, which is due to identifiable disorders. It also identifies levels of hypertension ranging from borderline (140/90) to uncontrolled (170/110). Hagberg (1988) also identifies "isolated systolic hypertension" to be especially common in the older adult population. It is found in only 1% of the population under 45 but occurs in 1/3 of the population 75 and over. With a blood pressure reading of 160 or more/ 95, it indicates difficulty in the ejection phase of the cardiac cycle. This may be related to the decreased arterial elasticity common to older adults, which results in increased resistance during the systolic (ejection) phase (Hagberg, 1988).

Benefits of Exercise

A gradual rise in blood pressure associated with aging appears to be largely connected to an increasingly inactive life-style. Studies demonstrate that endurance exercise produces a significant decrease in both diastolic and systolic blood pressure (Goldberg & Hagberg, 1990). Medicine-induced declines in blood pressure to the same levels produced by regular endurance exercise are associated with a 20% to 60% decline in mortality and morbidity. The additional benefit of exercise is its positive effect on the reduction of other risk factors associated with cardiovascular disease (Hagberg, 1988).

Exercise Modifications

The cardiac response to exercise in a hypertensive population varies according to the level of hypertension, medication, and individual differences. The evidence is clear, however, that high intensity exercise should be discouraged (ACSM, 1991a, b; Hagberg, 1988). A low to moderate level (40%–65% of maximum heart rate) at least 4 times a week appears to be very beneficial. Studies indicate that low intensity exercise at 50% of VO_2max (the highest volume of oxygen a person can consume during heavy exercise) actually results in a greater decline in systolic blood pressure (20 mm vs. 9 mm Hg) than higher intensity programs (Goldberg & Hagberg, 1990). Low- to moderate-intensity exercise therefore contributes to reducing blood pressure while putting the hypertensive exerciser at a much lower risk for cardiac difficulties.

Isometric contraction exercises (in which the muscle is strongly contracted without movement of the joint) are shown to increase systolic and diastolic blood pressure and therefore are not the best choice for hypertensive individuals. Exercises such as weight lifting which provide significant benefits in other areas can be approached with caution by utilizing low resistance with high (minimum of 20) repetitions (ACSM, 1991a). In weight lifting, proper breathing should also be stressed in order to prevent the increase in blood pressure that occurs if a person holds their breath while exercising against resistance.

Medication

Wilmore (1988) observes that beta-adrenergic blocking drugs (beta blockers) are among the most widely prescribed medications. They are regularly used for treatment of hypertension and coronary artery disease. Beta blockers can cause a modification of the heart rate of 15 to 60 beats per minute, depending on the dosage and the individual's responsiveness. Evidence further indicates that there is an increase in stroke volume in almost direct proportion to the decrease in heart rate, which allows cardiac output to remain nearly the same (Wilmore, 1988). There are a variety of beta-blocking medications that have varying effects; some affect cardiac response by limiting the heart rate, some are vasodilators, which decrease peripheral resistance in the blood vessels, and some affect both (ACSM, 1991a).

Several studies show that beta blockers may decrease the capacity for prolonged endurance exercise (Goldberg & Hagberg, 1990; Wilmore, 1988). This may have implications in the duration of aerobic exercise appropriate for the hypertensive individual. Other studies indicate that beta blockers may also have a negative effect on thermoregulation making those on such medication more susceptible to temperature extremes (Wilmore, 1988). Thus it is important to avoid having hypertensive individuals exercise in extreme heat, which would produce increased stress on the cardiovascular system.

The time exercise is performed in relation to when the medication is taken is also a significant factor. The body's response to exercise will vary according to how close exercise is performed to the peak response time (i.e., when the drug is having its maximum effect) (ACSM, 1991a). It is important to be aware of this factor in relation to formal exercise testing. For example, if exercise is normally performed 1 hour after taking the medication, then an exercise test should also be performed 1 hour after taking medication. In addition, as a senior exercise instructor it is essential that you relay to your medicated participants the significance of when medication is taken in relation to the performance of exercise. Consistent timing between medication and exercise will help ensure a more accurate assessment of the rate of perceived exertion by the exerciser. Because beta blockers artificially regulate the heart rate, medicated exercisers must learn to accurately assess their rate of perceived exertion during exercise. These individuals should not be trying to achieve a target heart rate determined by the Karvonen formula, because their medication invalidates target heart rate calculations.

CARDIOVASCULAR AND PULMONARY DISEASE

Cardiovascular disease is the leading cause of disability and death in the United States. Many older adults will exhibit some form of cardiovascular disease resulting from a variety of risk factors involving heredity and life-style. Cardiovascular disease is a broad term that can refer to a wide range of disorders of the cardiovascular system. Pulmonary disease relates to disorders affecting the respiratory system, including emphysema, bronchitis, and asthma. All cardiac and pulmonary disease has some implications for exercise programming, especially that involving aerobic conditioning.

Benefits of Exercise

Exercise helps to prevent heart disease and is also an important aspect of recovery from the functional losses resulting from heart disease. Heart attack survivors will begin their recovery in cardiac rehabilitation programs connected to hospital settings which facilitate the careful monitoring of exercise intensity and response necessary in this population. An older adult with pulmonary dysfunction can also benefit from exercise. Although regular exercise may not provide a significant increase in pulmonary function, it will help decrease respiratory symptoms. Involvement in regular exercise has also been shown to decrease anxiety and depression and improve one's ability to perform activities of daily living (ACSM, 1991b).

Exercise Modifications

A community-based senior exercise program focusing on low- to moderate-intensity exercise may be appropriate for heart patients in the final stages of recovery. However, such individuals should only participate in aerobic exercise under the careful guidance of their physicians, who will determine the appropriate level of exercise intensity and monitor their progress periodically. Those with pulmonary dysfunction must also modify the duration and frequency of exercise to allow for respiratory restrictions. For example, if 20 to 30 minutes of continuous exercise is unattainable, two 10- to 15-minute exercise sessions or even four 5-minute sessions may be appropriate (ACSM, 1991b). Even when exercise must be modified considerably from the ideal for optimal fitness, it is beneficial and should be pursued by those with cardiovascular and pulmonary disorders.

MUSCULOSKELETAL DYSFUNCTION

There are several musculoskeletal conditions common to an older adult population that significantly affect exercise potential and safety. These conditions can be disease-related, such as arthritis and osteoporosis, or involve an injury of a bone, joint, ligament, or muscle. They can also be due to chronic disuse.

Arthritis

According to the *Arthritis Foundation–YMCA Program Manual*, the word *arthritis* means joint inflammation and refers to a host of rheumatic diseases. Inflammation is characterized by swelling, pain, stiffness, and redness and can occur to varying degrees in the joints, muscles, and connective tissues of the body. Arthritis significantly limits the range of motion in the joints. It is considered a chronic condition (i.e., one having no cure) but can be managed through proper treatment programs.

Osteoarthritis is a progressive, irreversible form of arthritis characterized by degeneration of the articular surfaces of the joint. It usually involves continuous discomfort and affects weight-bearing joints, such as knees, hips, and spine. It begins most often after age 40.

Rheumatoid arthritis is a common inflammatory arthritis that can cause severe damage and usually affects many joints. It involves periods of acute pain during "flare-ups" and periods of little or no pain during "remission." It can occur at any age and more commonly affects women (ACSM, 1991b).

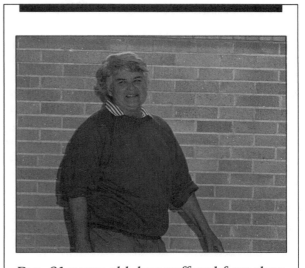

Bev, 61 years old, has suffered from rheumatoid arthritis for the past 13 years. This excerpt from a letter she wrote expresses what the arthritis water exercise has done for her: "After spending over 2 years trying every medicine known without positive results, I wound up in a wheelchair. Then I discovered water exercise when I came to live with my daughter who happened to be teaching for the Bozeman Young at Heart program. It truly was a turning point in my life. In 6 weeks I was out of the wheelchair. When I thought I was doing pretty well I moved back to my own town, but unfortunately there was no water exercise program there. Within 2 months I was back in the wheelchair. It was at that point that I knew that water exercise was always going to be a part of my life. I sold my home and moved to Bozeman to become a permanent fixture in the arthritis water exercise program, improving my physical function to a point where I can work 4 days a week.

Bev had a setback when a car accident caused a severe case of whiplash and other back injuries that prevented her from attending classes for almost a year. When she called to tell me that she was finally going to be able to start classes again, she talked about how great it was going to feel to get back in the water and regain her strength and mobility, lose the weight she had gained through the inability to exercise, and bring her arthritis back into check. "These classes are my lifeline," she says.

Benefits of Exercise

Arthritis is a major crippler in the United States, afflicting at least 30 million people and severely disabling an estimated 4.4 million (Pardini, 1987). Fortunately, exercise can have a significant impact on controlling the symptoms of arthritis. The proper types of regular exercise can help maintain a level of function in the joints that will allow those with arthritis to remain independent.

Exercise Modifications

It is important to include both range-of-motion and strength exercises in classes designed for those with arthritis. Strengthening exercises can include isotonic resistive exercise (in which the joint is exercising against light weight or some other resistance) or isometric exercise (in which the muscle contracts but does not move the joint). These types of exercise can safely and effectively improve strength, whereas vigorous exercise, which aggravates inflammation in the joints, is harmful.

According to the *Arthritis Foundation–YMCA Program Manual*, if a person has exercise-induced pain in the joints that lasts 2 hours or more after exercise, he or she has done too much. Exercisers must learn to recognize their own levels of ability and stop before signs of fatigue appear. Pain in the joint is a warning that the exerciser may be causing further damage to the joints. It is especially critical to adjust exercise during the occasion of arthritic flare-ups. Some flare-ups may require bed rest, passive exercise (someone else gently moving the joint through a range of motion), and direct physician supervision.

Non-weight-bearing exercise, such as water exercise, swimming, chair exercise, and cycling, are well tolerated by those with arthritis. While developing exercise sequences, alternate more difficult activities with easier ones to minimize fatigue. Encourage class participants to plan ahead for exercise class by not overexerting themselves before class. In addition, continually emphasize the importance of each person working at his or her own level of ability. Avoid the use of positions that can lead to joint deformity, such as tight grips on objects or the side of the pool during water exercise. Finally, weigh the risks to the joint with the benefits provided by the movement. For example, though a weight added to the ankle during knee extensions will increase muscle strength, it significantly stresses an already compromised knee joint; thus it is a contraindicated exercise for those with arthritis.

Two good resources dealing specifically with arthritis and exercise are the *Arthritis Foundation–YMCA Aquatic Program*, YMCA Program Store, P.O. Box 5076, Champaign, IL 61825-5076, (800) 747-0089, and *The Arthritis Exercise Book*, Cornerstone Library, Simon & Schuster Building, 1230 Avenue of the Americas, New York, NY 10020.

Osteoporosis

Osteoporosis in the older adult population is of significant concern, accounting for close to 1.3 million fractures a year in the United States. The highest incidence of fractures are vertebral at 550,000 a year, followed by hip fractures at 225,000 a year (Goldberg & Hagberg, 1990). By age 65, one third of women will have had vertebral fractures. By age 81, one third of women and one sixth of men will have suffered a hip fracture, which is often catastrophic and many times fatal (Rowe & Kahn, 1987). Osteoporosis is the loss of bone mineral density to such a degree that fractures can occur after even minimal trauma. Comparisons of a healthy bone and an osteoporotic bone are illustrated in Figure 2.3.

The main contributing factors to osteoporosis are the average decline of bone mass associated with the aging skeletal system, the elevated decline of bone loss due to the onset of menopause in women, heredity, and lifestyle factors (smoking, alcohol consumption, poor nutrition, and lack of physical activity) (Rowe & Kahn, 1987; Smith & Gilligan, 1989). Damage to the skeletal structure caused by osteoporosis cannot be reversed, so the only alternative is prevention of fractures or treatment of symptoms caused by fractures. There are currently three common avenues of prevention: estrogen replacement therapy for postmenopausal women, calcium supplementation, and increased physical activity (Smith & Gilligan, 1989). Studies done on young, amenorrheic (nonmenstruating) female athletes demonstrate that estrogen plays the largest role in preventing the decline in

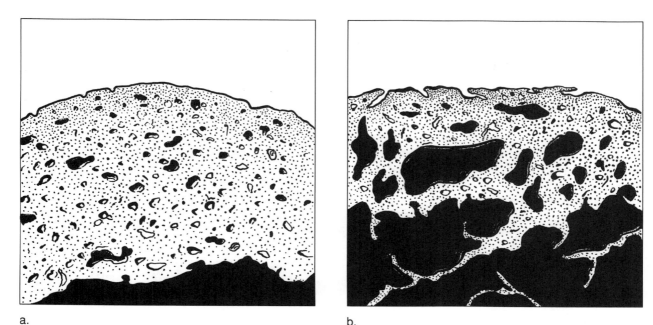

a.   b.

Figure 2.3 Comparison of normal (a) and osteoporotic (b) bone.

bone mineral density, with calcium and physical activity being important additions to the treatment.

Benefits of Exercise

Studies have shown that decreased activity promotes bone loss. Smith and Gilligan (1989) report that the removal or decrease of muscular or gravitational forces on bone segments causes bone atrophy. The degree of atrophy is influenced by the bone's normal role in weight bearing with those bones responsible for greater loads showing more rapid atrophy when the load is removed. Also, increases in bone mineral density are greater in the bones where the force is applied; for example, tennis players often experience significant bone hypertrophy (enlargement) in the dominant arm (Smith & Gilligan, 1989).

The most common study group for determining the effect of physical activity on bone loss intervention is postmenopausal women. This group is predisposed to osteoporosis due to the increased decline in bone loss associated with the loss of estrogen. Studies show that women in this study group who exercise regularly will slow bone loss and even gain bone mineral density (Goldberg & Hagberg, 1990). Other studies show that when formerly sedentary subjects participate in a regular physical activity program, bone loss is decreased or bone

mineral density is actually increased (Smith & Gilligan, 1989). It is also clear that when exercise is diminished, the loss of bone mineral density resumes.

Besides the obvious physical benefits, exercise appears to enhance one's feeling of well-being and may contribute to changes in other risk factors, such as poor nutrition. For example, exercise often stimulates one's appetite, which may result in improved nutritional intake (Smith & Gilligan, 1989).

Exercise Modifications

Research clearly shows that in order to affect the loss of bone mineral density, exercise must be weight bearing. Exercise that helps maintain muscle may also be beneficial, because those with greater muscle mass are less prone to osteoporosis than those with smaller muscle mass (Goldberg & Hagberg, 1990). Exercise for prevention of osteoporosis can be moderate-intensity, weight-bearing activities, such as low-impact aerobics and vigorous walking. Avoid ballistic or jarring movements. Also, some positions such as standing for extended times on one leg may place a vulnerable bone at risk. Such exercises should be limited to a maximum of 8 repetitions at a time. For those people who are in the later stages of osteoporosis, exercising while standing on one leg should be avoided completely.

Consider carefully the benefits versus the risks of any vigorous movements. For someone with osteoporosis who is at a high risk of falling, chair exercise and chair-assisted exercise would be more appropriate. One study on minimizing the detrimental effects of bed rest supports the idea that chair-assisted exercise may provide some benefits. Smith and Gilligan (1989) reported that even quiet standing helped slow the decline of bone mineral density associated with the total inactivity of bed rest. Also, when programming exercise for osteoporotic individuals, avoid excessive flexion of the spine (i.e., bending forward at the waist), which can contribute to spinal fractures and will place internal organs (already crowded due to osteoporotic-induced spinal changes) in a position vulnerable to injury.

Injury and Chronic Disuse Dysfunction

Some older adults will have a joint whose movement is compromised due to a severe injury of a muscle, tendon, or ligament. The injury may have occurred many years ago, and the affected muscles simply never received proper rehabilitation. In most cases, the muscle is no longer damaged but, due to disuse, will have lost the ability to function properly.

Others may suffer from dysfunction due to extreme muscle weakness caused by chronic disuse characteristic of a very sedentary lifestyle. Dysfunction caused by the extreme loss of muscle mass is common among those who have been ill and therefore chair- or bedridden for an extended period of time. Still, in most cases of injury or disuse dysfunction, proper exercise can significantly increase the function of the affected joint or muscle.

In the case of an injury dysfunction, a physical therapist is the best resource for determining what types of movements are appropriate for the affected joint and muscle segment. With the right kinds of movement, it may be possible to restore a greater level of function even when the injury is many years old. Exercises that involve some passive movement aid may be beneficial. For example, resistance bands, described in the chair-exercise portion of chapter 4, can also be used to aid the affected muscles in completing range-of-motion exercises.

In extreme cases of muscle weakness or loss of muscle mass due to chronic disuse, seek the advice of a physical therapist. In such cases, the joints can be very unstable due to the probable inflexibility of the tendons and ligaments that surround the joints and the weakness of the muscle tissues that would normally protect the integrity of the joint. The wrong kinds of exercises can pose an unacceptable risk of injury to this weakened structure. Once a physical therapist prescribes the types of movements that are appropriate, you can help your exercise participants accomplish the movement tasks in a variety of ways.

MEDICATIONS AND EXERCISE

In an older adult population, you will be dealing with people who are taking one or more long-term medications. It is important that you be aware of the kinds of medication your participants are taking, the potential side effects, and the possible interactions of combined medications. The effects of medication on exercise are as varied as the numbers of medications and the spectrum of individual reactions to medications. It is important, therefore, to make your participants aware of their responsibility in assessing—with their physician— the impact of their medications on exercise safety. It is imperative that you seek the advice of each participant's physician or pharmacist if you have any question about the safety of exercise and a specific medication. As a senior exercise instructor you must know what effects beta-blocker medications (used to treat hypertension) have on aerobic training. Also, be aware that many medications will affect sensory perception, balance, and coordination, so adhere to the guidelines in chapters 4 and 5 for providing safe movements.

PSYCHOLOGICAL AND SOCIAL ASPECTS OF AGING AND THE BENEFITS OF EXERCISE

Aging in our society is often accompanied by depression, feelings of isolation, and social detachment. Psychological factors can play a significant role in the decline of physical health even in the absence of any obvious physiological reasons. Berger (1989) concluded that psychological factors are one of the most significant predictors of both optimum health and longevity.

Loss of self-esteem is a common response in older adults to the attitudes surrounding advanced age in our currently youth-oriented society. A significant loss of self-worth often results in depression (Anspaugh et al., 1989). Depression is worsened by the emotional issues the older adult is likely to face—failing health, loss of family and friends, and financial problems (Berger, 1989).

Other psychological factors linked with aging include the need for maintaining autonomy and control and the importance of a network of social support. These issues have a close relationship to quality of life for older adults. Studies indicate that losses in autonomy and control are strongly linked to a decline in feelings of well-being, whereas the existence of a network of social support has a positive effect on both mortality risk and adherence to prescribed medical treatments (Rowe & Kahn, 1987).

Regular exercise can contribute significantly to improved self-concept, locus of control, and body image and decrease levels of anxiety (MacRae, 1986). Physical activity is consistently linked to enhanced mental health. Berger (1989) showed that exercise helps decrease the physical burdens of aging and thus enhances psychological well-being. According to Berger, exercise also reduces depression and promotes self-esteem, self-concept, and a positive body image. By attending regular exercise classes, the elderly can adapt to new social roles and establish ties with other members of their age group. Exercise is one of many worthwhile, enjoyable activities that can replace work responsibility after retirement and be an essential element for maintaining feelings of accomplishment and productivity.

Exercise also allows older adults to maintain their physical capacities, which in turn allow them to maintain an independent life-style, contributing significantly to happiness and self-efficacy (the belief that one is capable of performing a variety of tasks). Self-efficacy, in return, promotes feelings of competency and power and contributes to a higher level of physical activity (Berger, 1989). Maintaining an independent life-style is essential to maintaining feelings of autonomy and control, which are strongly linked to a feeling of well-being (Rowe & Kahn, 1987). This strong correlation between physical activity and life satisfaction illustrates the very close connection between physical and mental health.

CHAPTER

3

Meeting the Needs of Older Exercisers

Meeting the special needs of a senior exercise group requires attention to many details. You must consider the general components of your individual classes and carefully examine the safety issues of programming for older adults. In addition you must strive to develop a well-rounded program that addresses both the physical and the social and emotional components so important to a senior exercise program.

GENERAL PROGRAM COMPONENTS

The first step in programming exercise for seniors is to give special consideration to those components that form the foundation of any class—the instructor's role, proper scheduling, appropriate format, and the use of appropriate music. Attention given to these will help

you build a program that will meet the needs of this special population.

INSTRUCTOR

One of the most important elements to the success of any exercise program is the instructor. It is critical that an exercise leader be committed to safety as the highest priority. A senior exercise instructor must be properly educated in and have at least certifications in cardiopulmonary resuscitation and first aid. Additional certifications, such as lifeguard or emergency water safety, are required for water exercise if the pool does not have a lifeguard on duty during class time.

Generally, it is best to have a physical education or health-related background that allows you a depth of knowledge concerning the body's response to exercise. However, if you have not had formal education in this area, a reputable exercise instructor certification program will help you gain the necessary overview of vital information. It is also important to have some specialized training specific to senior exercise.

There are currently several programs that deal specifically with senior exercise. Time spent in education here will mean the difference between having a safe program *designed* for seniors or just having a modified low-level aerobics class. Write Kay Van Norman at Young at Heart, Department of Health and Human Development, Montana State University, Bozeman, MT 59717 or phone her at (406) 994-6316 for information on bringing a senior exercise instructor training workshop to your location. You can choose from a series of half-day, full-day, or 2-day workshops including programs on principles of senior exercise, chair exercise, basic exercise, low-impact aerobics, resistance training, water aerobics, arthritis water exercise, using self-directed poster programs, modifying line and folk dances for seniors, and adding fun and variety to your senior classes. Here are other senior exercise resources available through the Bozeman Young at Heart program:

- A beginning level chair exercise videotape (appropriate for senior citizen centers, residence facilities, or in-home use)
- Senior exercise poster programs (different sets for different ability levels, focusing on maintaining functional fitness).
- Senior resistance training poster programs (utilizing stretchy bands and light weights)
- Senior-specific visual aids (rate of perceived exertion chart and land-based and water-based heart rate charts)

Here also is a list of other reputable programs that provide information on senior exercise. Those with an asterisk are programs that offer some form of instructor training.

*American Alliance for Health, Physical Education, Recreation and Dance
Council on Aging and Adult Development
1900 Association Drive
Reston VA 22091

*Arthritis Foundation–YMCA Aquatic Program
Available through
    YMCA Program Store
    P.O. Box 5076
    Champaign IL 61825-5076
    Phone: (800) 747-0089

*Mary Mayta
Life International
PO Box 11528
Wichita KS 67202

*Dorothy Chrisman
Body Recall
PO Box 412
Berea KY 40403
Phone: (606) 986-2181

Mary Ann Wilson
Sit and Be Fit
2428 East 39th
Spokane WA 99223

Dee Ann Birkel
School of Physical Education
Ball State University
Muncie, IN 47306

Many seniors will also rely heavily on their exercise instructor as a health resource. It is important that you are well informed on the latest information in exercise and other health-related areas but equally important that you do not step past the bounds of your knowledge. It is not unusual for class participants to ask you to confirm or rebuke their doctor's advice in a variety of areas. Contradicting a doctor's advice in a health matter poses an unacceptable safety and liability risk.

Besides being well educated in the special needs of seniors, you must care about the individual seniors in your program. The relationship between instructor and students in a successful seniors' class is personal and caring. Be friendly, upbeat, and ready to hug, touch, and be personal. Most senior students will want to know about you as a person, your family, and your interests.

They also will want you to know them. Take the time to get to know your students. Many seniors will come to class 15 to 20 minutes early to warm up by walking and visiting with others. This is an excellent time to learn about your students. It is also a good idea to allow 5 to 10 minutes to answer questions or just visit with individuals *after* class. And be sure to contact students who suddenly stop attending to see if they are well. Most seniors will appreciate a call to check on their well-being and will be pleased to note that they were missed.

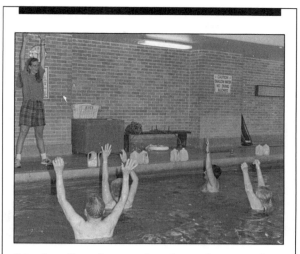

I took a few days going from class to class to ask the seniors what qualities they like to see in an exercise instructor." "Enthusiasm," June says. "Yes," Alice agrees, "we need someone who can motivate us to move by making class fun."

"They also need to be willing to do the exercises with us because in the pool it is difficult to hear instructions; many times we just follow along with what the instructor is doing on the pool deck."

"And they need to perform the exercises in the right order," Minnie says, "starting slowly and working up to the more difficult aerobics, then giving a good cool-down."

"I like it when instructors walk around the pool area and watch each person," June adds. "Then you know they care if you are doing the exercises properly."

Enthusiasm and being fun to exercise with also rank high in the low-impact aerobics class. "I like an instructor who can get me motivated on those days that I have a hard time getting up and getting to class," Elsie says. "When the instructor is enthusiastic it makes me glad I made the effort to get here, and when class is over I know the day's off to a good start."

"I appreciate an instructor who uses good music and keeps rhythm with the music," Norma says.

"And someone who keeps us moving and gives us a good workout," Bob adds.

They all agree wholeheartedly: As long as they are putting in the time, they like to get a good workout!

It is also important that you make an effort to help your senior exercisers to get to know and interact with each other. Social interaction during class time will encourage students to develop a new network of "exercise friends" that will likely carry over into their daily lives. This more personal atmosphere between instructor and student and student and student gradually develops a bond of trust and respect within the class and becomes an important reason why seniors continue to attend.

SCHEDULING CLASSES

The morning hours are generally the most popular for senior exercise classes. Many seniors are very busy with volunteer work and club activities, which are usually scheduled in the afternoon. Then, too, they come from a generation that learned "early to bed, early to rise . . . ." The hours of 8, 9, and 10 in the morning seem to be the most popular; 7 a.m. can also be a popular hour, especially in the summer months. More important than the particular hour is that the time is scheduled and *consistent*. Do not assume that because many seniors are "retired" that any time is satisfactory. Their involvement in volunteer work, clubs, and other organizations means that classes must be scheduled on consistent days and times each week.

It is also best to stay in one location. Most senior students like to be comfortable in familiar surroundings, so a seniors' class that bounces from one place to the next is likely to have a difficult time building up a following. Exercising at one location will also allow effective use of bulletin boards or other information centers. An information center is a good way to promote a feeling of comfort and familiarity. A stop at a bulletin board that regularly provides health information, recipes, even jokes and keeps everyone informed of program events and schedule updates will soon become a regular part of the class routine.

CLASS FORMAT

Several formats can be effective for senior classes. The standard 1-hour format with 10 to 20 minutes of warm-up, 20 to 30 minutes of aerobics, and 15 to 20 minutes of cool-down and stretching works well (refer to chapter 4 for

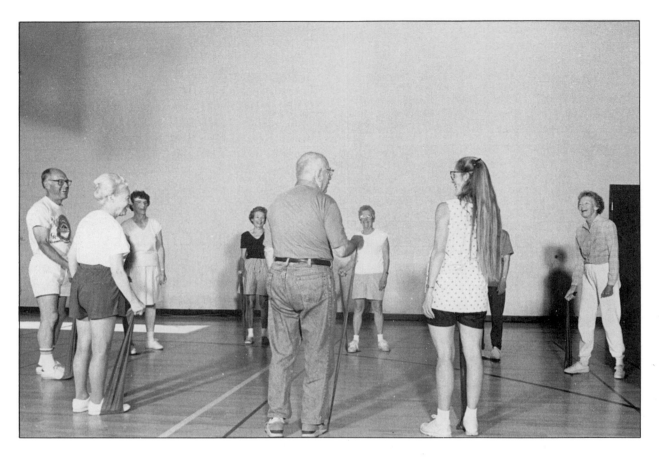

Encourage students to make "exercise friends" through social interaction in class.

specific exercises). Classes for beginners will have longer phases for the warm-up and the cool-down and stretching. As the class becomes more fit you may increase the time spent doing aerobics, and some of the warm-ups can approach low-level aerobics. Always, however, maintain at least 10 minutes of warm-up and 15 minutes of cool-down and stretching. Allowing seniors to perform aerobic exercise without proper warm-up and cool-down can pose health risks for them and liability risks for your program.

You also should give special consideration to making time for a social aspect in an exercise program for seniors. The warm-up and cool-down phases lend themselves well to allowing social interaction while moving.

If you are housed in a fitness facility with access to weight machines and other special equipment, such as stationary bikes, you may want to use a 90-minute "stations" format. For example, you could offer 30 minutes of warm-up of choice (stationary bike, walking, light weight

training) followed by 30 minutes of aerobics of choice (water or low-impact exercise, stair climber, stationary bike); and then 30 minutes of cool-down and stretching (t'ai chi, yoga, floor work, water-based stretching). Implementing this type of format will require careful explanation of the required phases (warm-up, aerobics, cool-down) and monitoring of individual progress to ensure that students are achieving the proper balance. It also poses challenges in maintaining the social aspect, especially group cohesion. You may want to do at least one phase of the class, such as the cool-down, as a group. While developing a flexible program that makes use of the equipment available to you, also take the time to plan forums for social interaction.

This social component is of vital importance to a seniors' class and is a strong motivator for continuing to come to class. It is ideal if you have a place where students can come early or stay late to sit and visit, have a cup of coffee or juice, and generally feel at home and part of something special. If not, then you must

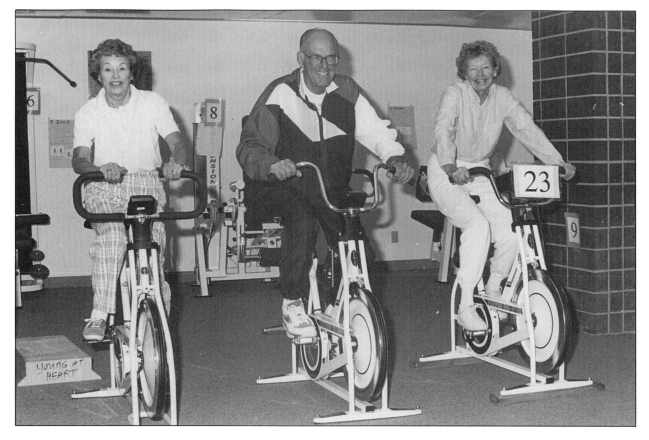

Plan your class format according to the facilities and equipment you have available.

designate class time for interaction. Warm-ups or cool-downs done in a circle and in partners will help facilitate conversation. Maintaining a friendly banter throughout the class so all feel free to talk will also promote a sense of belonging among participants.

MUSIC

Music plays a significant role in the success of a senior exercise class, so be sure that the music you choose contributes to participants' overall enjoyment. The music must be age-appropriate—music that participants can relate to and feel comfortable with. Imagine walking into an aerobics class filled with college students and using Frank Sinatra and Glenn Miller songs for the whole class. The idea of using the current Top 40 hits in a seniors' class is just as ridiculous, and it will yield the same results—an unenthusiastic group today, and an empty room next session. Using music popular with the senior generation will have them

singing along, reminiscing, and truly enjoying their time in class.

Choose music that has distinct rhythm without overpowering vocals; midrange vocals with simple instrumental accompaniment and clearly understood words work well. Instrumentals with a distinct continuous rhythm are another good choice, but avoid those with excessive embellishment of the melody—the rhythm may get lost in embellishment and become difficult for senior exercisers to follow. Be aware, too, that music with very high instrumental or vocal notes can be torturous for people who wear hearing aids.

You don't need to restrict your music selections only to "oldies" tunes; popular songs can be used as well. Look for songs that are pleasant to listen to or sing along with, have vocals in the midrange, and are fun and upbeat for aerobics or slow and relaxing for cool-down. Try new songs between "oldies" and watch reactions. Then ask your students which songs they liked. Don't worry, most seniors are not afraid to give an opinion if you ask them. Use

Warm-up and Cool-down

Max ByGraves	Midrange vocals for warm-up and cool-down
Glenn Miller	Big band vocal and instrumental selections for warm-up and cool-down
John Denver	Midrange vocals for warm-up and cool-down
George Winston	Nice instrumental piano selections for cool-down and relaxation
Mark Knopfler	"Princess Bride" soundtrack; instrumental relaxation
Ray Lynch	Nice instrumentals for warm-ups, especially "Deep Breakfast" and "Celestial Soda Pop"

Aerobics

Max ByGraves	Midrange vocals, many in 3 to 4 song medleys such as "Won't You Come Home Bill Bailey?" and "Bye, Bye Blackbird" (order from record store)
Herb Alpert	Many moderate tempo instrumental selections, like "Spanish Flea," "Sentimental Over You"
Glenn Miller	Many moderate tempo selections, vocals and instrumental, like "In The Mood," Chattanooga Choo Choo," "Chattanooga Shoe Shine Boy"
Roger Miller	Midrange vocals, like "Engine #9," "England Swings," "King of the Road"

Broadway show tunes, such as "Hello Dolly" and "Cabaret"

"Hooked on Classics" I, II, & III—Royal Philharmonic Orchestra instrumental medleys

"Hooked on Swing"—Manhattan Swing Orchestra instrumental medleys

music that you also enjoy as this will promote your own enthusiasm. Refer to the above list for age-appropriate musical suggestions to use in your senior exercise classes.

In addition to the right type of music, consideration must also be given to the appropriate volume. Many senior students have hearing difficulties. Some will be partially corrected by hearing aids, but others will be completely uncorrected. This does *not* mean turn the music up louder! Most seniors dislike loud music, and those who have some degree of deafness will not necessarily benefit from the increased volume. In most cases, they will be straining to hear your instructions, and loud music will only make this more difficult. Seniors with hearing aids will be most troubled by loud music because the aid magnifies all sounds, which produces an uncomfortable and irritating jumble of music, voices, and background noises. So, play music at a modest volume and watch to see how your seniors are responding to the music. Ask them if they can hear the *rhythm* and if they would like an adjustment in the volume. It won't be long before you can easily recognize the appropriate volume for your particular class.

SAFETY

Safety must be the number one priority in senior exercise classes. With other age groups, aerobic conditioning may be the top priority with safety an important secondary concern.

However, in a senior exercise class, you are dealing with a population that has a very high incidence of coronary artery disease, high blood pressure, heart disease, osteoporosis, arthritis, and muscle and joint dysfunction. Senior students can be at risk for heart attacks, strokes, joint and muscle injuries, and fractures. Many seniors also have significant deficiencies in balance, coordination, and strength that can pose a high risk of falling. In addition, sensory impairments, such as low vision or hearing, or medications that affect depth perception and reaction time can add to the risk.

To manage all of these risks, apply your foundation knowledge of exercise science and age-related functional ability to all aspects of your senior exercise class. Provide a thorough warm-up, carefully monitor aerobic exercise intensity, and ensure a proper cool-down to allow your seniors adequate time to recover from the aerobic phase before they leave your class. In addition, give careful consideration to the physical conditions common to the senior population that require special exercise modifications. Remember always to weigh the risks with the benefits of *all* movement choices to ensure safer programming for senior exercisers.

MANAGING AEROBIC TRAINING AND MOVEMENT RISKS

To monitor the aerobic phase, you must calculate each student's target heart rate zone and then do frequent heart rate checks. Train your students to evaluate their own rates of perceived exertion and use this guideline in conjunction with the target heart rate guidelines. Get to know your participants so you will notice if they look or act differently than normal, and be alert to any sudden change of behavior or appearance. *Never* allow a participant to leave class without a proper cool-down. If someone has to leave class early, have him or her stop the aerobics session a little early and walk around the space until his or her heart rate drops well below the aerobic training zone. If someone leaves class unexpectedly, have an assistant or another senior follow to determine if the person is experiencing a health problem.

Make sure you have the proper training to respond to an emergency, and regularly practice emergency procedures with your class.

Besides careful monitoring of exercise intensity, consideration must be given to managing movement risks. When choosing exercises, always weigh the risks with the benefits for each movement. In all types of exercises for seniors, avoid jerky or ballistic movements that can stress the joints and muscles. In land-based aerobics, avoid high risk movements such as quick footwork with surprise changes of direction that could cause ankle turns, trips, and falls. Remember that the diminished levels of strength, balance, and coordination (which in some cases are exaggerated by sensory impairments) pose a high risk of falling.

Also, remember that a high percentage of your female senior participants will suffer from varying degrees of osteoporosis and therefore will be at a high risk for fractures. Many older adults who sustain a hip fracture will end up in long-term care and of those, approximately one half will die within 1 year. Obviously, because of the overwhelming risks, fancy footwork such as fast cross-over steps or surprise direction changes do not meet the standards for safe senior exercise.

ENVIRONMENTAL RISKS

Be aware of environmental hazards. For example, a hot room is unsafe for aerobic conditioning for seniors. Those with high blood pressure are at greater risk of cardiac problems when they become overheated. If senior exercisers become red-faced, perspire significantly, or mention how hot the room feels, it is too hot! As the exercise leader, be sensitive to how your own body temperature is responding to exercise; this will help alert you to signs of excessive heat in your students. If the room cannot be better ventilated or the room temperature lowered, do not attempt aerobic conditioning.

In contrast, a room that is too cool will make it difficult to adequately warm up before aerobic movement. Older adults generally have less flexible muscle, tendon, and ligament fibers, so a cold room can significantly decrease their ability to warm up properly and increase their risk of muscle pulls and strains. A room is too cold if you or your students feel chilled during the warm-up and experience an uncomfortably rapid cool-down after the aerobic phase. It is very difficult to provide a proper (i.e., gradual) cool-down and safe stretching for seniors in a cold room.

Besides the temperature of the environment, also pay attention to the surface your class will be exercising on. Look for slick, sticky, or uneven spots on the floor. Remember a fall or trip can mean embarrassment and a bruise to the younger exerciser but a possibly life-threatening fracture to many older adults. See chapter 6 for more specific information on appropriate environments for your senior exercise program.

MINIMIZING LIABILITY

Liability is a topic of concern for any exercise class, but it is of special concern in this high-risk field. For your protection and the protection of your participants, you *must* require that participants seek a physician's consultation before they start your exercise program. The liability/waiver forms that you use must ask specific questions about high blood pressure, heart disease, coronary artery disease, osteoporosis, arthritis, any cardiovascular abnormalities, and medications currently used. Many people will neglect to include important information unless it is specifically requested (see Figure 3.1 for a sample liability form). There are also good sample liability forms provided in *Mature Stuff* published by the American Alliance for Health, Physical Education, Recreation and Dance. (Be aware that even a signed waiver of liability will not protect you from a lawsuit if you act in a negligent manner.)

Take the time to interview new participants concerning their past and present activity levels, so you can make informed recommendations for the type and duration of exercise in which they can safely participate. This will also help you guide participants in developing realistic goals and make them more aware of the importance of proper exercise intensity. Update the liability information for your regulars yearly to keep you informed of any changes in their health status.

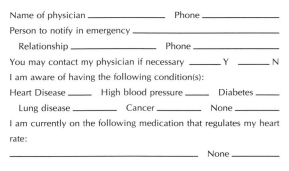

Figure 3.1 Sample liability form.

EMERGENCY PROCEDURES

A well-rehearsed emergency plan is essential. This plan must involve all of the steps necessary to care for an injured or ill individual and to summon medical help. In the case of an emergency during class, it will likely be a senior participant who calls for emergency personnel while you provide care to the injured party. Therefore, post all emergency procedures next to the phone using large, high contrast print readable by the average senior (e.g., black print on white paper). Readability is even more critical for water exercise classes in which senior participants will likely not be wearing their glasses.

In addition, each instructor should have a list of the students in class, including information on the medical condition of each student (taken from the liability forms). This will help the instructor and emergency personnel deal effectively with the situation.

Rehearse all emergency procedures with your instructors and your classes on a regular basis so that everyone involved is confident of the procedures. Seniors are well aware of the possibility of illness or injury during exercise and will be more comfortable knowing that there is a solid workable plan for such emergencies.

PROVIDING A WELL-ROUNDED EXERCISE PROGRAM

To meet the needs of your target population a well-rounded seniors' exercise program must provide safe movements and involve as many of the basic components of fitness for your particular group as possible. When choosing movement possibilities, *always* weigh the risks against the benefits of each type of exercise. Choose smooth rather than jerky arm movements and "completed" movements rather than choppy or jerky starts and stops. Also use low-impact movements that keep at least one foot in contact with the floor at all times, coupled with simple movement patterns. Smooth, completed movements reduce the risk of joint stress and injury to senior participants. In land-based exercise classes, low-impact movements are the only correct choice for seniors, because high-impact movements pose a very high risk of injury. Simple movements and movement combinations are also safer and promote self-confidence by allowing the participants success in movement. Many seniors have lost some degree of coordination, especially if they have not been regularly participating in a coordination-promoting activity. For this reason rapid changes of direction and complicated movement patterns increase both the anxiety of the participants and the danger of falling. They also decrease self-esteem and enjoyment for those who are unsuccessful in executing the movement.

The need for simple movement poses the extra challenge for you, the instructor, to come up with an interesting variety of movement combinations, music, and teaching formations. Vary the basic front-facing formation by using circles, lines, and partner groupings. (Such varied formations also facilitate social interaction. There are many folk dances that can be simplified to meet safety guidelines and still add a great deal of fun and social interaction to classes (see chapter 4 for specific exercises).

WARM-UPS

Combine continuous movement with gentle range-of-motion activities and easy strengthening work for your warm-up. *Never* start a senior exercise class with stretching. Seniors tend to have relatively stiff, inflexible tendons, ligaments, and muscles, which means a higher potential for muscle and tendon strain or tear. Instead, begin the class with gentle, continuous movement, such as walking, smooth movement to music, or easy range-of-motion activities to increase circulation.

If you plan to use a new sequence of movements in the aerobic phase of a class, the warm-up is a good time to teach the sequence. This will give the students a chance to move slowly and gain confidence before trying to execute the movement in time to music.

During the warm-up, take your students through the range of motions they will be performing during the aerobics section. For example, if you plan to push the arms overhead during the aerobic phase, then perform the same action slowly during the warm-up. Save the stretching to increase range of motion until *after* the aerobics phase, when the body is warm.

AEROBICS

Due to the high incidence of cardiovascular dysfunction in the older adult population, you must use a variety of methods to help ensure that your participants are exercising at an appropriate aerobic level. The key to a safe aerobic component in your senior exercise program is careful determination and monitoring of exercise intensity.

Determining Exercise Intensity

Seniors need cardiovascular conditioning to maintain and improve function, but it must be

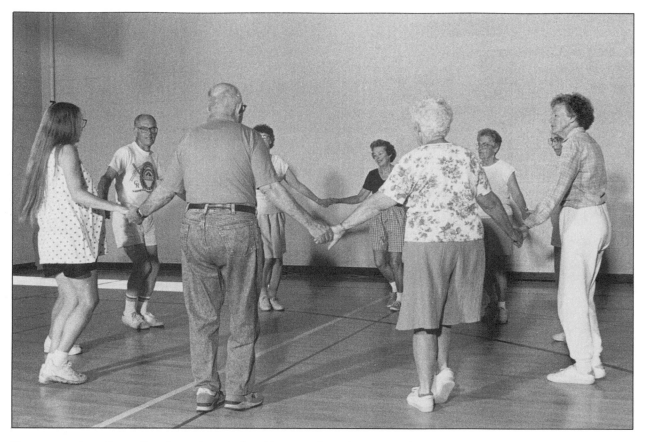

Vary your class formation by using circles, lines, and partner groupings.

at a safe level that allows slow, gradual improvement. This can be achieved through the determination of safe, individual target heart rate zones, use of the rate of perceived exertion, and frequent heart rate checks. It is also important to learn the signs of possible overexertion, such as rapid breathing, loss of coordination, and flushed skin. By using this combination of methods, you can help your students discover exactly how intense their exercise should be.

Target Heart Rates

Safe, individual target heart rate zones can be determined using the Karvonen formula, which incorporates each participant's age and resting heart rate. However, it is unnecessary—and unwise—to let your seniors attempt to reach a level of 80% of their maximum heart rate, which is the standard high range of this formula. Research shows that even moderate- to low-intensity aerobic exercise provides a training benefit for many seniors. A safe level for senior students without heart disease would be from 50% at the low end to 75% at

the high end (see Figure 3.2 for the senior-modified Karvonen formula). Make certain that all seniors know their target heart rates and what their 10-second counts should be.

Those senior students with known heart disease should be exercising at a heart rate recommended by their physicians and by their rates of perceived exertion. Note that *heart rate medications invalidate target heart rate calculations*, so you must know which of your students take medication that necessitates use of the rate of perceived exertion instead of Karvonen's formula to determine their exercise intensity. Even for your nonmedicated students, using the rate of perceived exertion coupled with the modified Karvonen's formula to determine exercise intensity adds another welcome measure of safety to the aerobic component of class.

Rate of Perceived Exertion

Many medications artificially regulate the heart rate and thus invalidate target heart rate calculations. Therefore, students on these

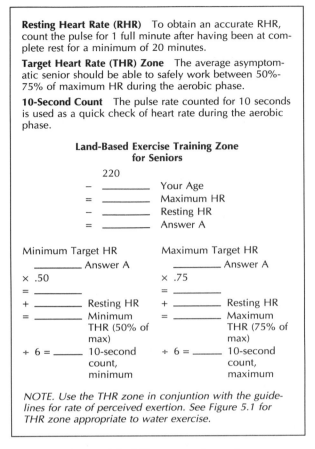

Resting Heart Rate (RHR) To obtain an accurate RHR, count the pulse for 1 full minute after having been at complete rest for a minimum of 20 minutes.

Target Heart Rate (THR) Zone The average asymptomatic senior should be able to safely work between 50%-75% of maximum HR during the aerobic phase.

10-Second Count The pulse rate counted for 10 seconds is used as a quick check of heart rate during the aerobic phase.

Figure 3.2 Modified Karvonen formula.

Modified rate of perceived exertion		
	1	very, very light
	2	very light
	3	moderately light
SAFE ZONE	4	light
	5	moderate
	6	moderately hard
	7	hard
DANGER ZONE	8	very hard
	9	very, very hard
	10	extremely hard

Figure 3.3 Modified rate of perceived exertion.

medications must not try to achieve a predetermined heart rate. Instead, they should rely on assessing their own rate of perceived exertion, which gauges how an individual feels during and after exercise.

There are a variety of scientific rate-of-perceived-exertion charts with numbers corresponding to target heart rates. However, a simple, straightforward chart like the one in Figure 3.3 is best. A color-coded chart, numbered from 1 (light) to 10 (hard), effectively relays in a simple, nonthreatening manner the concept of "how hard do I feel I am working." The color coding can indicate the moderate range exercisers should try to achieve and warn against working in the hard range.

Even for those participants *not* on heart rate medications, the rate of perceived exertion provides important information about how they are responding to exercise *that day*. The body's response to exercise is affected by many things, such as heat, cold, medications, stress, or slight illness. Because of these (and other) factors, individuals may actually be exercising below their target zones but feel like they are working hard. Giving the rate of perceived exertion equal importance to the calculated target heart rate zone will help ensure that participants are exercising at a safe level in line with their bodies' response to exercise that day.

Standing Resting Heart Rate

Instead of calculating individual target heart rate zones, some programs use a guideline of approximately 20 beats above the participants' "standing resting heart rate." The standing resting heart rate is a person's heart rate when he or she walks into class that day. This heart rate can vary dramatically depending on what the person encountered while getting to class, so it is best to have a specific planned activity before taking the pulse. Slowly walking around the space then doing some slow, even breathing and relaxation movements would be a good choice. Using the standing resting heart rate plus 20 beats as a guideline for the aerobics is a safe alternative to computing target heart rate training zones, so long as it is used in conjunction with the rate of perceived exertion.

Monitoring Exercise Intensity

Monitoring exercise intensity takes very little time but gives you important feedback on how your students are responding to exercise. Using a variety of techniques, both objective and subjective, will significantly increase the safety of your program.

To improve the reliability of heart rate checks, your method of checking the heart rate must be simple and consistent, so that all class members can successfully find and count their own pulse. Use the same cues each time you take an exercise pulse rate. Make the cues clear and direct: "Stop and find your pulse" (pause for 2–3 seconds); "Ready, start" (count for 10 seconds); "Stop." As soon as the 10-second count is completed, the participants can begin marching in place while each person tells you her or his 10-second count. Practice taking exercise pulse and recovery pulse rates with your students so they all feel comfortable with and confident about doing the procedure, and each heart rate check will only take a few moments.

There is some discussion of whether it is better to take the pulse at the carotid artery on the neck or at the brachial artery on the wrist. Due to varying levels of diminished feeling in the tips of the fingers, many seniors will have difficulty finding and counting their pulse. Therefore have them try *both* the carotid and the brachial pulse points to determine which one works best for them.

The carotid pulse should be taken by placing the fingers of the right hand onto the right side of the neck close to the windpipe. Caution your students *not* to press too firmly on this spot— too much pressure could cause a person to become lightheaded. Also tell them to avoid reaching across the throat to the right side of the neck with the left hand or grasping at the windpipe area with the fingers on one side and the thumb on the other (and thus squeezing the windpipe). Both of these positions can restrict the flow of oxygen and cause participants to become lightheaded.

The brachial pulse should be taken by placing the fingers (*not* the thumb) of the left hand onto the "thumb side" of the front of the right wrist (palm facing up). Firm pressure here will not cause a problem. Take the time to make sure that all students can successfully find their pulses at one location or the other. If you rush through this procedure, it is likely that a higher percentage of your seniors will not

actually take an accurate heart rate reading but will simply call out a number similar to the ones they hear around them. This can pose a danger because it sidesteps one of your primary methods of ensuring proper exercise intensity.

During the aerobic phase, have students practice determining their rates of perceived exertion by asking each person to give you a number that indicates how hard each feels that he or she is working according to the rate-of-perceived-exertion chart (see Figure 3.3). By requiring each individual to make this determination, you reemphasize the importance of proper exercise intensity and the probability of differences between individuals in their response to exercise. It will also help those students who have difficulty finding and counting their pulse to find an exercise intensity that feels comfortable.

Frequent Heart Rate Checks

During each class period, check heart rates after the warm-up. This will tell your seniors how their bodies are responding to exercise that day. Then continue to monitor exercise intensity frequently by checking heart rates 2 or 3 times during the aerobic phase and asking each person his or her 10-second count. Ask those seniors on medication that artificially regulate the heart rate, such as beta blockers, for their rates of perceived exertion. This frequent checking will alert you immediately to any potential problems.

At the end of the aerobic phase, check their exercise heart rates again. Have everyone walk slowly for 1 minute and then take their own recovery pulse for 10 seconds. Ask students how many beats they decreased in the 1-minute recovery period. If you have students whose pulse rates do not decrease after 1 minute, take their pulse again 1 minute later to determine if it has decreased. Failure of the heart to recover noticeably after aerobic exercise can be an indication of a variety of problems. Such individuals should be monitored throughout the rest of the class to determine whether their heart rates are responding. A senior whose heart rate goes overly high (heart rate 12 to 15 beats over their maximum target heart rate) and who does not recover promptly should be referred to his or her physician.

Before beginning the cool-down phase, again ask students, regardless of whether they are on heart rate medication, to indicate their rates of perceived exertion. This will help your students become aware of how they feel when they are exercising within their own target heart rate zones.

Recording Exercise Intensity

For easy referral, write your students' predetermined 10-second counts or some mark indicating their reliance on the rate of perceived exertion next to their names on a role sheet or chart. Keep a record of each student's exercise heart rate, recovery heart rate, and rate of perceived exertion for every exercise period during the first several weeks of class (see the sample chart in Figure 3.4). Recording these figures will help you to become familiar with each individual's response to exercise and alert you to any potential problems, such as excessively high exercise heart rates or failure of the heart to recover after 1 minute. It will also help reinforce to your students the importance of monitoring exercise intensity with both the target heart rate and the rate of perceived exertion. After you become familiar with your class

members and their responses to exercise, continue to ask each participant for these numbers even if you no longer take the time to record them.

FLEXIBILITY

Flexibility is just as important to seniors as aerobic conditioning. Maintaining flexibility is critical to functional fitness, the level of fitness necessary for individuals to take care of their personal needs, maintain an independent lifestyle, and continue to participate in activities that they value. The ability to live independently is of critical importance to seniors and is a chief prerequisite to enjoying a positive quality of life. Therefore, when you design work for flexibility, consider how it contributes to functional fitness by helping maintain range of motion in all joints and promoting ease of movement. Make "movement that matters" your motto as an instructor. Think about the bending, stretching, and reaching that are

Date														
Name	EHR/R	RPE	EHR/R	RPE	EHR/R	RPE	EHR/R	RPE	EHR/R	RPE	EHR/R	RPE	EHR/R	RPE

EHR = Exercise heart rate; R = Recovery heart rate; RPE = Rate of Perceived Exertion

Figure 3.4 Sample record-keeping chart.

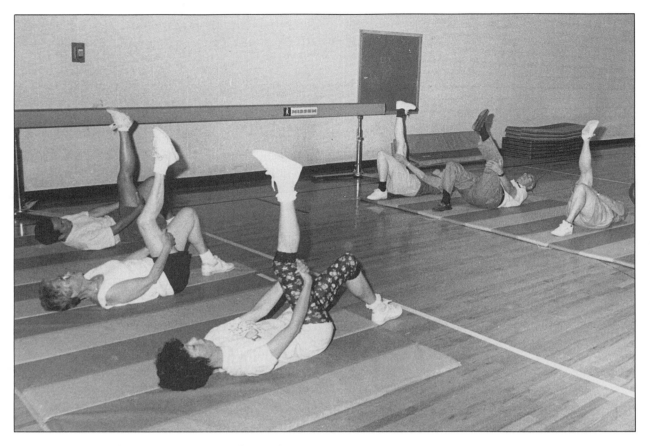

Relax while stretching to protect muscles and joints.

necessary in any given day to maintain an independent life-style and prevent loss of function: These are movements that matter.

Give special attention to the areas that are typically troublesome for seniors—the upper back, neck and shoulders, lower back, and hamstrings. Gentle, slow stretches are the only ones that are appropriate for seniors. You must also take into account that there is a high incidence of muscle and joint dysfunction among the senior population, so it is important to offer alternative exercises or modifications for many stretches. Protect the joints by keeping the body relaxed as much as possible while stretching a particular muscle group (see chapter 4 for land-based stretches and chapter 5 for water-based stretching).

STRENGTH

Many seniors have a significantly diminished level of strength. This especially holds true for older women. Research indicates that a large percentage of women aged 55 and over cannot successfully lift and carry 10 pounds. Considering all of the things that a person must lift and carry in the course of a day, strength plays a large role in functional fitness. It also helps to prevent injury to joints and to maintain balance and prevent near falls. This is of critical importance as falls are listed as the third highest cause of accidental death among seniors (ODPHP, 1990).

Strength work should be slow, smooth, simple movement for both the lower and upper body. Take special care to protect the joints through proper alignment, and carefully weigh the risks against the benefits of each movement. Whenever possible, incorporate strength work into your classes by using rubber bands, stretchy bands, small weights, or water resistance. Light weight lifting for many repetitions (e.g., 8–15 reps) using free weights or machines will achieve good results with seniors. Weight lifting is a great confidence builder, because it achieves rapid, readily noticeable results.

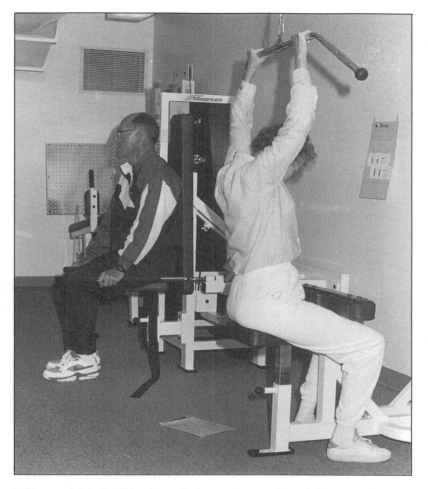

Lifting weights builds strength in seniors and contributes to functional fitness.

COORDINATION AND BALANCE

Coordination and balance are two very important factors in maintaining functional fitness. Both play a large role in the prevention of falls and can deteriorate rapidly, if not exercised. Coordination can be easily addressed in the class through unison and opposition work, sequencing of movements, and an endless variety of arm and leg combinations. Balance activities are more easily done in the water (which reduces participants' fear of falling), rising onto toes, transferring weight to one foot while lifting the other off the pool bottom, or rocking forward onto the toes and back onto the heels. In land-based exercise, balance work can be done standing in circles, holding hands for support, or standing next to a wall.

Practicing balance and coordination will increase your senior participants' confidence in movement. It will also provide opportunities for increased self-esteem as, with practice, the balance and coordination activities become progressively easier to perform.

SOCIAL AND EMOTIONAL COMPONENTS

The emotional and social component contributes significantly to the success of any senior exercise program. When programs that successfully meet the exercise needs of seniors fail to provide their need for emotional and social interaction, they stagnate. On the other hand, programs that seem to focus on this aspect, though lacking in some important exercise components, gather more and more participants in spite of the deficiencies. In any case, it is the instructor who sets the atmosphere of the class and is ultimately responsible for facilitating its emotional and social aspects.

SOCIAL INTERACTION

Social contact with others is consistently one of the top five answers to the question I ask in my program, "Why do you come to the senior exercise class?" For many senior participants, exercise class may be the highlight of their day. It is a place they are expected to be, an appointment, somewhere to meet with others of their own age with similar interests, a place where they are a significant part of a group.

The members of an exercise class become a unique support system for each other. For example, those who have lost spouses can resocialize themselves in exercise classes. For many widows and widowers, their longtime friends are generally still couples, which can make them feel like "third wheels" at social gatherings. Thus, it is very important that they find an additional network of support, a place where they "fit in." An exercise class can provide that network. Carpooling to class, taking part in activities before or after class, and planning to socialize outside of class all help expand the exercise participant's support network.

In addition, senior exercisers know that if they don't show up for class, others will be asking about them and likely calling to check on them. A primary concern—even fear—of many seniors who live alone is that they will fall or otherwise be incapacitated and not be found for many days. Knowing that others are watching out for them is a tremendous benefit of being a regular part of an exercise group.

Make a point of devoting some time in each class to social interaction. This can be as simple as exercising in a circle, which allows participants an opportunity for friendly exchanges. You can also have a designated time during warm-up or cool-down when you converse with the students and encourage interaction. Simple social mixer dances and activities can introduce new participants, help everyone learn each others' names, and ensure that everyone is involved in the fun. When the students become comfortable as a group, an activity such as the shoulder circle rub (see photo on p. 39) is a great way to facilitate talking and laughing—and it feels great!

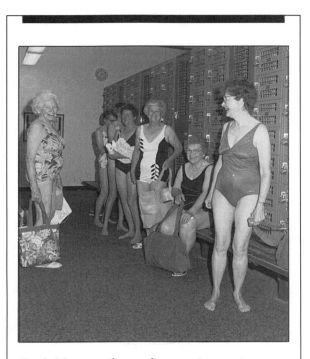

By 6:30 a.m., the early morning water exercisers are dressed and ready a good 1/2 hour before their 7 a.m. class, lined up on the benches talking and laughing. Many in this group have been attending the same early morning class (7 a.m. in the summer, 8 a.m. the rest of the year) for 6 years. Asked the standard question about what keeps them coming to water exercise, "Arthritis," says Minnie. "If I wasn't exercising, I would barely be able to move." "It just makes me feel good," says Anne. The others agree. When asked why they get here so early, they look at each other and chuckle. "It's easier to find a parking place if you get here early," June says. They come up with other sensible reasons, such as not liking to hurry to get dressed and allowing plenty of time in case they have car problems. Then Mary says, "When you have exercised with the same people for 5 to 6 years, you get kind of attached to them." Helen laughs, "We have lots of visiting to get done, and you can't do that in class while you're concentrating on the exercises." The smiles and nods confirm that this social interaction with people they have grown to care about is the real reason they can be found perched on the benches in the locker room long before class begins.

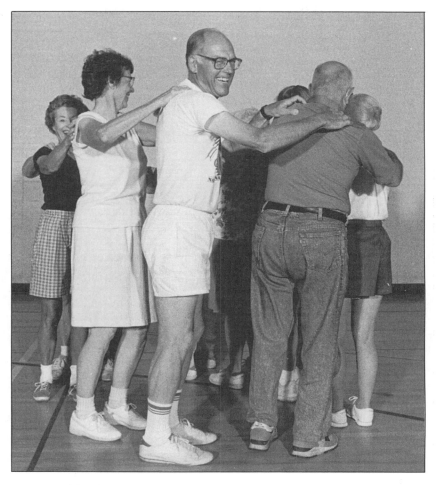

Activities like the shoulder circle rub promote class interaction while helping students loosen up.

SELF-ESTEEM

Success and enjoyment in movement in a positive, noncompetitive environment significantly contribute to increased self-esteem. Providing an opportunity for a feeling of accomplishment and success in movement is an essential element of a senior exercise class. Make a special effort to ensure senior participants that they can all be successful movers in your class. Everyone wants to feel as if they can successfully perform the exercises and exercise combinations in a class—especially seniors. Many of your senior students will not have exercised in a group setting for many years, possibly since grade school. They may come into your class thinking that they probably can't keep up. If you reinforce that idea, they will walk away with a confirmation that "I am not capable of fitness exercise." Your job is to make sure they are successful in movement. Avoid complex combinations and complicated steps. Use simple movement patterns and easy-to-follow rhythmic patterns. Provide a noncompetitive environment in which everyone is encouraged to work at their own levels, and frequently demonstrate variations appropriate to different levels of ability. Give positive reinforcement for all accomplishments and efforts. Have a simple "home-base" step, such as marching in place, that everyone can perform easily and return to it frequently. A home-base step before and after a new movement gives each participant a chance to be successful a large percentage of the time and provides a positive exercise experience. Feeling at ease in performing movement to music will also increase self-esteem and promote a feeling of accomplishment.

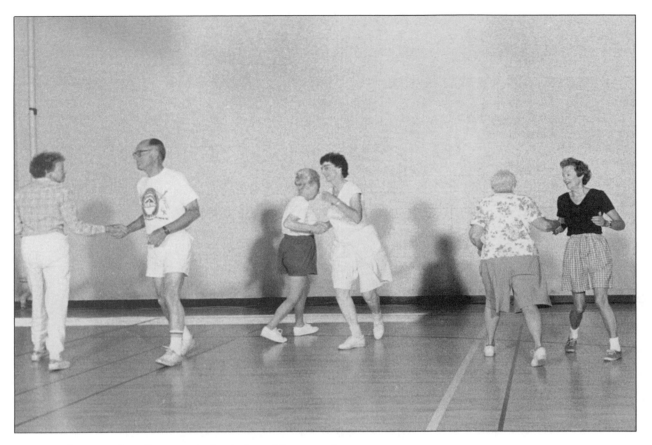

Build self-esteem by allowing students to achieve regular success.

Once your senior participants feel successful, then you can offer them additional challenges like more complex patterns interspersed with a simple home-base movement, such as marching in place. Challenges met with success further increase self-esteem and encourage confidence when facing other challenges, not only in exercise but in other areas of life. Remember: Always balance challenge with ensured success, and always weigh the benefits against the risks for all movements.

CHAPTER

4

Land-Based Programming

In a land-based exercise program you can develop a range of classes designed to meet the needs of a variety of levels of functional ability. This chapter focuses on programming chair exercise for the somewhat restricted or very sedentary senior, basic exercise for the mildly restricted or healthy but sedentary senior, and low-impact aerobics for the healthy, active senior.

Regardless of the level, class should begin the moment your seniors enter the room. Many will come early to walk around the space or sit and visit with the other participants and the instructor in a "pre" warm-up, both physical and mental. Making this time before class a priority contributes significantly to the social and emotional component of your program. Greet everyone and welcome them to class. If there are new participants, introduce them to the group and to individuals and ask a long-time member to act as their "sponsor." This will help newcomers immediately feel like a part of the group.

CHAIR EXERCISE

Chair exercise can vary in intensity from vigorous chair aerobics designed to gain aerobic training benefits for the healthy senior to movement that concentrates on maintaining a minimum level of function in the muscles and joints of the frail elderly. In this chapter I will address the middle level of chair exercise, consisting of a combination of chair exercise and chair assisted exercise designed to improve range of motion, strength, coordination, and balance. It also provides an opportunity for socialization and fun. The target population for mid-level chair exercise is the somewhat physically restricted senior with joint problems that prevent ease in walking, cardiovascular or respiratory disease that precludes participation in any aerobic activity, or the chair bound. The following resources can give you more information on the various levels of chair exercise and help you fit your program to your target population.

Frail elderly
Charlie Daniel
HPER Department
Western Kentucky
Bowling Green, KY
42101

Mid level
Kay Van Norman
Young at Heart
Dept. of Health
  & Human Dev.
Montana State University
Bozeman, MT 59717

Low to mid level
Mary Ann Wilson, RN
Sit and Be Fit
2418 East 39th
Spokane, WA 99223

Low to high level
Eva Montee
1433 N.E. Loucks Rd.
Madras, OR 97741

CAUTIONS

Because of the likelihood of a high incidence of osteoporosis among those attending your chair exercise class, there are certain movements you should avoid or use sparingly. Avoid all jerky, ballistic movements and rapid twisting or turning of any body part. Also, avoid excessive compression of the abdominal area, especially for those participants who show evidence of an osteoporotic spine. Bending all the way over at the waist can put stress on internal organs that may already be crowded, due to spinal fractures and the resulting compression and forward curvature of the spine. Similarly, standing on one leg exerts a great deal of pressure on what may be an osteoporotic, and thus dramatically weakened, hip joint. To protect the hip joint, avoid standing on one leg for more than 8 counts, and avoid any twisting motion of the hip while standing on one leg.

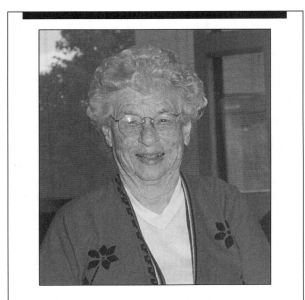

Bertha Clow at age 91 shares some thoughts on exercise. "I am a member of the chair exercise class and I never miss," she says proudly. "I think that I really need the exercise to keep going as many years as possible." Bertha recently broke her hip in a fall in her apartment at the retirement facility. I went to visit her in the hospital, where she was in good spirits. Her hip had been repaired and she was able to get up and walk with a walker. She said that she was grateful the chair exercise was available to her right where she lived and she was really looking forward to getting back to class in a couple of weeks. "The doctor says that I am doing very well, and I know it's because I have continued to exercise," she added.

MOVEMENT THAT MATTERS

When planning your class, focus on *movement that matters* by identifying those movements that seniors should be able to perform easily in order to take care of their own personal needs. Include exercises that improve strength in the quadriceps muscles, which allow them to rise up from and lower down onto chairs, get into and out of bed, and go to the toilet without assistance. Include upper body mobility exercises to help participants maintain the ability to comb their own hair, dress themselves, and otherwise take care of their personal needs. Emphasize exercises that strengthen the upper back to help maintain an upright posture. Repeat each exercise 4 to 12 times, depending on the level of ability of your particular group.

Also, remember that it is important to maintain the ability to lift and carry things of various sizes and weights. Light resistance exercise with stretchy bands or 1-pound to 3-pound weights can improve strength. Talk to your class, find out which everyday activities they would like to be able to perform more easily, and then build a program that provides movement that matters.

SPECIFIC EXERCISES

To create a well-balanced exercise series, start from the top of the head and work down through the body, concentrating on moving each joint through its appropriate range of motion. Perform all exercises gently, completing the full range of movements slowly and smoothly. Routinely remind participants to keep breathing normally throughout all of the exercises with extra reminders to breath normally while holding a stretched position.

In the following exercises the *neutral* position is sitting up straight in the chair with the shoulders directly over the hips (the spine is *not* relaxed into the back of the chair), facing forward, shoulders square to front, arms hanging relaxed at the sides, head and neck centered, feet flat on the floor. All exercises begin in this neutral position, unless otherwise specified.

Neck Exercises

Caution: *Do not allow exercisers to lift the chin past neutral and drop the head back. This can cause cervical compression and dizziness. Avoid all rapid or jerky movements with the neck.*

▌ *Ear to Shoulder:* Exercisers gently lower right ear toward right shoulder, return to neutral; lower left ear toward left shoulder, return to neutral; then lower chin toward the chest, and return to neutral. Use a slow 8- to 12-count hold in each position. The shoulders should remain down in a relaxed position throughout the exercise.

▌ *Neck Rotation:* Participants look over right shoulder, return to neutral, look over the left shoulder, return to neutral, pull the chin back (keeping head level), return to neutral. Perform each movement to a slow 8 counts.

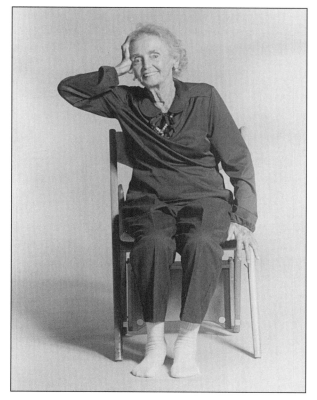

4.1 Neck stretch.

▌ *Neck Stretch:* With the palm of the right hand on the right side of head, exercisers use the neck muscles to push against the hand with the head for 4 to 8 counts (caution them not to hold their breath), then release the hand and relax the neck to neutral. Then gently drop the left ear to the left shoulder and hold for 8 counts; return to neutral. Repeat the exercise with the left palm on the left side of the head. See Photo 4.1.

▌ *Nose Circle:* Exercisers slowly draw small circles in the air with their noses 2 to 3 times clockwise, then 2 to 3 times counterclockwise (8 counts for each circle).

▌ *Pendulum:* Participants gently drop chin toward chest and draw a half circle on the chest by keeping the chin down and slowly rotating the head to the right, return to center, then rotate to the left (like a pendulum). Use 4 to 8 counts to complete each movement.

Shoulder and Upper Back Exercises

Caution: *Exercisers must avoid dropping the arms forcefully from a position above the head or out to the sides. After lifting the shoulders up, the return to neutral should be slow and controlled.*

▌ *Shoulder Shrugs:* Exercisers lift both shoulders to ears, return to neutral; press shoulders down, return to neutral. Use 4 counts for each movement.

▌ *Shoulder Lifts:* Participants lift right shoulders up, left shoulders up; right shoulders down, left shoulders down (1 count each). Then move both shoulders up, both shoulders down (2 counts each).

▌ *Shoulder Circles:* Exercisers move one shoulder (or both) in circular motion, forward or backward 4 to 8 counts for each circle.

▌ *Blade Squeeze:* Exercisers round shoulders forward (4 counts), return to neutral (4 counts); pull shoulders backward so shoulder blades squeeze together in back (hold for 8 counts), then return to neutral (4 counts).

■ ***Squeeze and Stretch:*** With hands on shoulders, elbows out, participants touch elbows together in front (4 counts), return to neutral (4 counts). Then press elbows toward back so that shoulder blades squeeze together (8 counts), and return to neutral (4 counts).

■ ***Arm Reaches:*** Using one or both arms in any combination with the hand(s) returning to touch the shoulders between each reach, exercisers reach out to sides, hand(s) to shoulders; reach overhead, hand(s) to shoulders; reach forward, hand(s) to shoulders; reach down, hand(s) to shoulders.

■ ***Cross Arm:*** Exercisers reach right arm across the front of the chest to the left, then hold the right forearm with the left hand and gently stretch (*not* jerk or tug) the right shoulder for 8 to 12 counts. Then they release the right arm and return to neutral (4 counts). Repeat the stretch with left arm crossing the chest to the right. See Photo 4.2.

Elbow, Wrist, and Hand Exercises

■ ***Biceps Curl:*** With hands on thighs palms facing up, exercisers flex the elbows and touch the hand(s) to the shoulders. Alternate right and left, or use both at the same time. To increase biceps strength, exercisers place the

left hand on the right forearm and push down, resisting the right biceps curl (see Photo 4.3), and repeat with the left arm (caution them not to hold their breath). A stretchy band or light weight may also be used for resistance. Avoid shoulder impingement by not allowing the elbows to get behind the body in any upper body strength moves that involve the shoulder joint.

■ ***Curl and Touch:*** With hands on thighs palms facing up, exercisers flex the right elbow touching the right hand to right shoulder, then touch the right hand to the left shoulder, touch the right hand again to the right shoulder, and return hand to thigh, palms facing up. Repeat using left hand (1 count for each movement). Finally, repeat the movement using both right and left hands at the same time.

Caution: *Alternate finger work with wrist work in order to prevent overstressing potentially inflamed joints.*

■ ***Prayer Hands:*** Exercisers press palms together in praying position (4 counts), slowly lift the elbows out to the sides until the wrists flex to approximately 90 degrees (4 counts), hold for 4 counts, then bring elbows down in 4 counts.

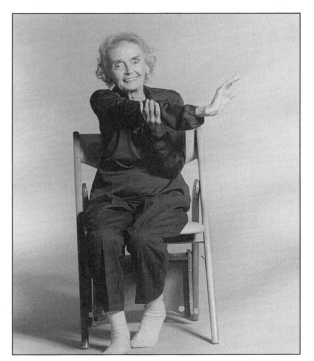

4.2 Cross arm.

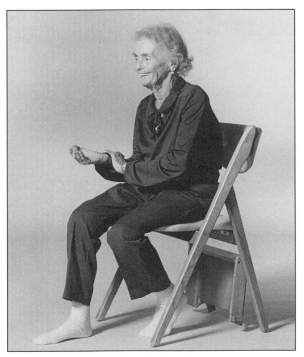

4.3 Biceps curl with resistance.

Wrist Circles: Exercisers slowly rotate wrist in circles, with open hands then with hands closed into fists.

Finger Fan: Exercisers close the hands to fists, open and spread the fingers apart, close extended fingers together like a fan, open and spread fingers apart, close fingers, then close the hands to fists (2-4 counts for each movement).

Finger Drawing: Exercisers draw circles in the air with one finger at a time on both hands (i.e., both thumbs; then index, middle, ring, pinky fingers). Alternate directions and utilize the full range of motion. For variety, exercisers may write names, addresses (etc.) in the air with each finger.

Finger Circles: Exercisers touch the index finger and thumb together to form a circle; repeat with each finger (1 count for each). Then they close the hands into fists (2 counts), and open and spread the fingers wide (2 counts).

Torso Exercises

All torso exercises should be done sitting up straight in the neutral position without dipping the shoulders to the right or left.

Torso Isolations: Exercisers shift the torso to the right side, return to neutral, shift to the left side, return to neutral (2 counts each); push torso to the front, return to neutral, pull to the back, return to neutral (2 counts each); then make a full circle right (8 counts) and a full circle left (8 counts).

Contraction: Exercisers round the back (but *not* by sinking down or slumping in their chairs) and press grasped hands forward for 8 counts; then slowly straighten the back while opening the arms out to sides then lowering them to the neutral position over 8 counts. See Photo 4.4.

Rotation: Exercisers gently turn to the right and, twisting at the waist, look over the right shoulder (turn 4 counts; hold 8 counts); return to neutral (4 counts); then repeat the movement to the left.

***

Caution: *Avoid forceful twisting from side to side. This exercise should be done gently and slowly.*

***

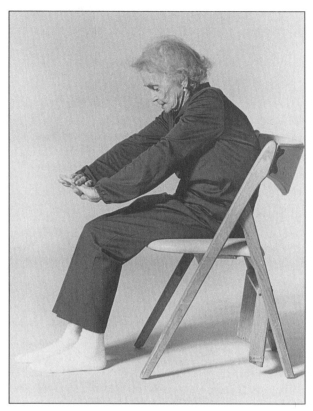

4.4 Contraction.

Reach and Pull: With right arm, exercisers reach as far across to the left side of the body as possible. Now tighten your arm muscles as if grasping something and pulling it toward yourself while returning your arm to neutral using 4 counts; then using the left arm, reach to the left and "grasp and pull" while returning to neutral. Repeat the movement toward the right with the left arm reaching across the right side of the body and pulling back to neutral, then the right arm reaching to the right and pulling back to neutral, again over 4 counts each.

***

Caution: *Be sure that the feet are flat on the floor at least shoulder-width apart while doing this exercise. This will prevent reaching over too far and losing balance.*

***

Deep Breaths: Exercisers take a deep breath, fully expanding the rib cage, then blow the air out evenly; repeat. Emphasize filling the lungs to their fullest capacity each time and then expelling air completely.

Hip Exercises

Exercises for the muscles that support the hip joint can be done in the neutral position, except the spine should be relaxed up against the back of the chair to allow for more freedom of movement in the hip socket.

▌ *Leg Cross:* Exercisers lift the right leg (knee bent) straight up center (Counts 1 and 2), cross it over the left knee (3, 4), bring back to center (5, 6), then return to neutral (7, 8); repeat with the left leg crossing right. See Photo 4.5.

▌ *Leg Open Side:* Exercisers lift the right leg (knee bent) up center (Counts 1 and 2), open to the right side (3, 4), close to center (5, 6), and return to neutral (7, 8); repeat with the left leg opening to the left side.

▌ *Hip Rotation:* Participants extend the right leg to the front with the foot flexed, rotate the leg out from the hip, and return to center, rotate in, and return to center. (This rotation will be small, so be sure it is occurring at the hip, not the knee or ankle.) Repeat 4 times before returning leg to neutral. Then repeat the whole series with the left leg. See Photo 4.6.

Caution: Instruct participants to keep the back straight while performing the following knee lifts.

▌ *Knee Lifts:* Exercisers do alternating knee lifts to the front, touching right hand to right knee, or do cross knee lifts touching the left elbow to the right knee and the right elbow to the left knee, 1 count for each movement. Return to neutral after each knee lift.

▌ *Double Knee Lifts:* Exercisers lift the right knee to the front, then return to neutral. Lift right knee to the front again, and return to neutral. Repeat, lifting the left knee 2 times.

▌ *Hip Stretch:* Exercisers carefully place the right ankle on the left knee, gently press down on the inside of the right knee to stretch the right hip (the right leg will be rotated to the right at the hip with the knee pointing to the side), hold the stretch for 8 counts, then return to neutral. Repeat the movement on the left side with the left ankle resting on the right knee. See Photo 4.7.

Caution: This exercise should not be done by anyone who feels tension or pain in the knee while in the stretched position.

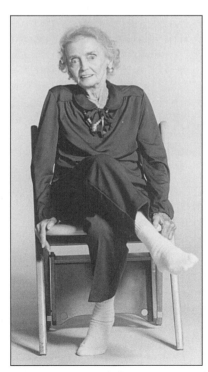

4.5 Leg cross.

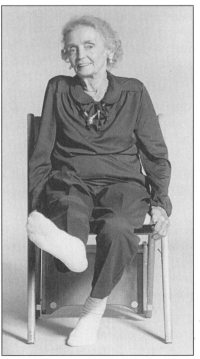

4.6 Hip rotation.

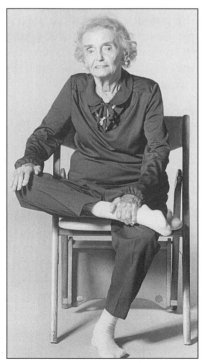

4.7 Hip stretch.

Knee, Ankle, and Feet Exercises

Caution: Whenever the legs are extended to the front be sure that participants keep their abdominal muscles engaged and backs straight with no hyperextension of the lower back.

▌*Knee Extensions:* Using 2 counts for each movement, participants extend the right leg to the front, then flex the knee back to neutral. Repeat 4 to 8 times right, repeat with the left leg. To promote quadriceps strength, have exercisers cross the left ankle over the right so that when the right leg is extending to the front, it is also lifting the weight of the left leg; repeat with the other leg.

▌*Extend and Point:* Exercisers extend the right leg to the front (Counts 1 and 2), point the toe (3, 4), flex the foot (5, 6), point (7, 8), flex (1-2), point (3-4), flex (5-6), return to neutral (7-8). Repeat with the left leg.

▌*Extend and Circle:* Participants extend the right leg to the front, perform right ankle circles in each direction utilizing the full range of motion (allow 8 counts for each circle), and return to neutral; repeat with the left leg. To promote quadriceps strength, increase the time that the leg remains extended to the front (e.g., do points, flexes, ankle circles, and pronation and supination of the foot) before returning to neutral.

▌*Ankle Rocks:* Exercisers raise up onto toes, then press the heels down to a flat foot; rock back onto both heels, pulling toes off the floor, then press toes down to a flat foot. Use 2 counts for each movement)

▌*Toe Curls:* Keeping the sole of the foot on the floor, exercisers do toe curls (i.e., grip the floor with the toes), return to neutral, pull toes up and back (off the floor), then return to neutral. Allow 2 counts for each movement).

▌*Toe Taps:* Keeping the heels on the floor, exercisers do alternating toe taps while flexing the ankle as far as possible each time (they will feel the contraction in the front of the shin), 1 count for each tap. Instead of alternating, participants may do up to 8 toe taps with the right foot before changing to the left.

Chair-Assisted Standing Exercises

There are three main positions for chair-assisted exercises: standing directly behind the chair with both hands on the chairback (neutral), standing to the right of the chair with the left hand on the chairback (right-side neutral), and standing to the left side of the chair with the right hand on the chairback (left-side neutral). The hands should only rest lightly on the chair. Caution your participants not to lean on the chair or rely solely on it for balance. See Photos 4.8 a, b, and c.

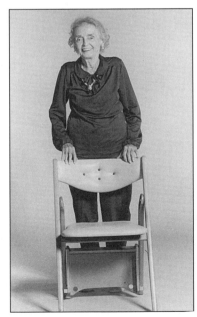

4.8a Neutral.

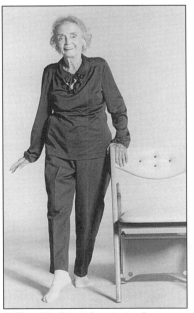

4.8b Right-side neutral.

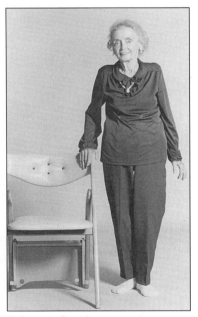

4.8c Left-side neutral.

▌ *Relevé:* Standing in neutral position, exercisers press up onto the toes (Counts 1 and 2), hold (3, 4, 5, 6), then bring heels down (7, 8).

▌ *Plié:* Standing in neutral position and keeping both feet flat on the floor, exercisers bend both knees (Counts 1 and 2), hold (3, 4, 5, 6), then straighten legs (7, 8). Participants should keep the back straight throughout the exercise and bend the knees directly over the toes.

▌ *Achilles Stretch:* In the left-leg-forward lunge position, exercisers press the right heel to the floor, hold for 8 to 12 counts, return to neutral. Repeat on the opposite side in right-leg-forward lunge position. See Photo 4.9.

▌ *Hamstring Contraction:* Standing in neutral position, exercisers contract the hamstring and gluteus muscles to flex the knee and lift the right heel toward the right buttock (Counts 1 and 2); hold (3, 4, 5, 6), then return to neutral (7, 8). Repeat, lifting the left heel toward the left buttock. This movement can be done as a double heel lift: Exercisers flex and lift the right heel 2 times, return to neutral position, flex and lift 2 times on the left, then return to neutral position.

▌ *Press Backs:* Beginning in neutral position, exercisers lift the right heel until the knee is flexed to 90 degrees (Counts 1 and 2), press the right leg back 2 times, keeping the knee flexed and the back straight (3, 4 and 5, 6), then return to neutral (7, 8). Repeat with the left leg. See Photo 4.10.

▌ *Touchouts:* Beginning in right-side neutral position, exercisers reach out with the right toe to touch front (Counts 1 and 2), as shown in Figure 4.8b, touch side (3, 4), touch back (5, 6), and return to neutral position (7, 8). Then bend the knees keeping heels on the floor (1, 2), straighten the legs (3, 4), bend knees (5, 6), straighten legs (7, 8). Repeat exercise on right except touch toe back, toe side, toe front, return to neutral position, bend knees, straighten, bend knees, straighten. Repeat the entire sequence using the left leg beginning in left-side neutral position.

Using Props

Props add interest, variety, and fun. There are many low-cost items that can be both beneficial and fun to use. You can make 1- to 3-

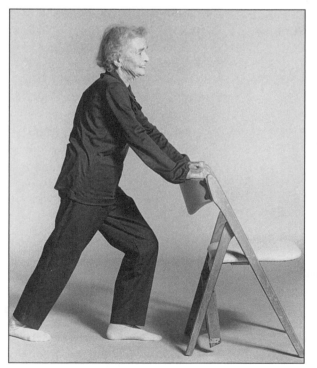

4.9 Achilles stretch.

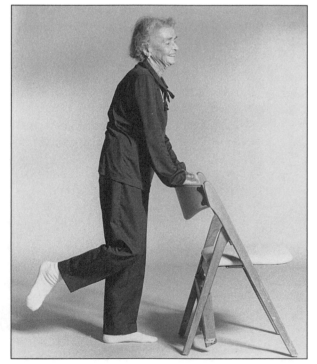

4.10 Press backs.

pound weights from PVC pipe and lead shot from a hardware store, or use large rubber bands from an office supply store, yarn balls, or homemade "Ping-Pong" paddles made from old nylons stretched over metal coat hangers. Look through books on elementary-school physical education programming for more ideas on making low-cost equipment. You will find that many common items can be used in your senior exercise classes—just use your imagination.

Kooshie Balls

Kooshie balls, found in many toy stores and large discount stores, are a wonderful prop for a chair-exercise class. They are light and easy to handle, have an interesting feel, and can be easily squeezed in one hand. Use them to exercise the hand and fingers. For example, try a variety of sequences such as squeeze 8 times right hand, 8 times left hand, 4 times right, 4 times left, 2 times right, 2 times left, 1 time right, 1 time left.

Kooshie balls are easy to toss up in the air and catch, because they will not bounce off a person's hands like a tennis or foam ball. To improve coordination, have participants toss the Kooshie up and clap one or two times before catching it again. Or use them in partner work where participants sit across from each other and toss 1 or 2 balls back and forth.

Kooshie balls rolled up and down the legs and arms and between the hands provide tactile stimulation and improve circulation. You can also use them to exercise the feet. Rolling them back and forth with the sole of the foot provides a wonderful foot massage (without shoes, of course). Participants can also attempt to pick the Kooshie ball up from the floor by gripping it with their toes.

Sponges

Sponges of various sizes and shapes can be squeezed, tossed, and gripped with the toes similar to Kooshie balls. Or squeeze large sponges placed under the arms to work the shoulder and upper arm muscles or between the knees to work the inner thigh muscles. Small sponges can be squeezed or wrung in the hands, or rolled and squeezed with the feet and toes. They can also be used in toss-and-catch games, though they bounce off the hands easily.

Wooden Dowels

Wooden dowels can be used as aids in stretching and strength-promoting exercises. For example, have participants hold the dowel in neutral position (horizontal to the floor in front of the body with both hands approximately 8-10 inches apart), raise the dowel to the shoulder level (Counts 1 and 2), push it over the head (3, 4), pull the dowel down behind the head (5, 6), hold (7, 8); push it back up over head (1, 2), pull down behind the head (3, 4), hold (5, 6), push up (7, 8); return to front shoulder level (1, 2) and then to neutral (3, 4), and rest (5, 6, 7, 8). Participants can exercise the wrists by turning the dowel forward or backward in their hands.

Standing exercises can also be done with dowels. Exercisers can use them like canes, placing one end down and strutting or even doing a step-kick sequence around it to vaudeville-type music. Use your imagination to come up with simple, safe routines.

Newspapers

Newspaper can help improve hand agility. Have each senior hold one sheet of newspaper by the corner with the right hand, then, using the fingers of the right hand only, wad the newspaper up into a ball. Next, have seniors transfer the newspaper ball into their left hands and then, using only the left hand, uncrumple the newspaper ball.

Resistance Bands

Resistance bands are made of a stretchy elastic type of material and come in a variety of strengths, from light resistance to heavy resistance. (The light- to medium-resistance bands are most appropriate for a chair-exercise group.) The two most common brands, Dynabands and Therabands, can be ordered from many fitness supply catalogs either precut or in bulk rolls that allow you to measure and cut the size of resistance band that meets your needs.

Resistance Band Exercises

Resistance bands can be used to develop both upper and lower body strength. When working on upper body strength, be sure your seniors keep the elbow next to or in front of, rather than behind, the body. Having the elbow behind the body while performing strength moves that involve the shoulder joint can create impingement of the shoulder joint, a painful condition for a senior exerciser. A strip of resistance band approximately 3 feet long works well for the following exercises.

▮ *Biceps Curl:* Exercisers place the right foot on one end of the band and grip the other end with the right hand, keeping the wrist locked straight (avoid hyperextending the wrist), then flex the elbow to bring the right hand to the right shoulder (biceps curl). Number of repetitions will depend on the strength of the participants and the resistance of the band (4-10 times is a good range). Repeat for the left arm. See Photo 4.11.

▮ *Chest Press:* Have seniors place the band behind the back at waist level and grasp one end with the right hand and the other end with the left hand. With elbows touching their sides, they slowly push their arms out to the front to extend the elbows, then slowly flex the elbows to bring them back to the starting position. Do not allow the elbows to go past the sides behind the back when returning to the starting position.

▮ *Triceps Press:* Grasp one end of the band with your left hand against your chest. Grasp the other end of the band with your right hand (6 to 8 inches from left hand). Keeping the right elbow just below shoulder level and the lower arm parallel to the floor, press the right hand forward, extending the elbow. Slowly, return to the starting position. Repeat 4 to 10 times, and then do the exercise sequence with the left arm. See Photo 4.12.

▮ *Upright Row:* With the right foot on one end of the band, exercisers grip the other end with the right hand, elbow extended straight down and palm facing back, then flex and raise the elbow to the side until the upper arm is parallel to the floor (no higher than shoulder level), lower slowly to a straight arm. Seniors should do 4-8 reps, then repeat the exercise using the left hand. See Photo 4.13.

▮ *Brake Push:* The exerciser places the left foot in the middle of the band and grasps one end with the right hand and one end with the left hand. She brings the left knee up toward the chest and pulls her elbows to the sides.

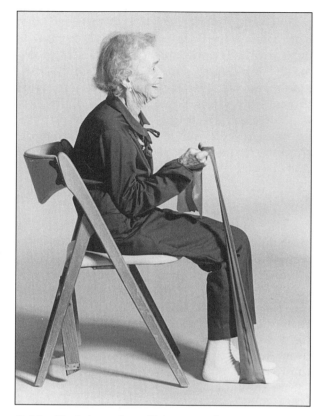

4.11 Resistance band biceps curl.

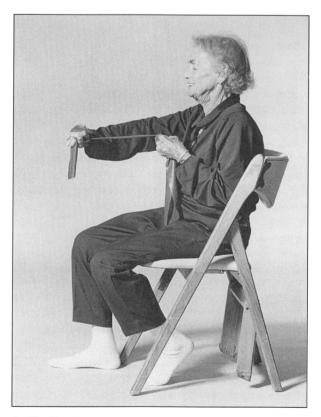

4.12 Triceps press.

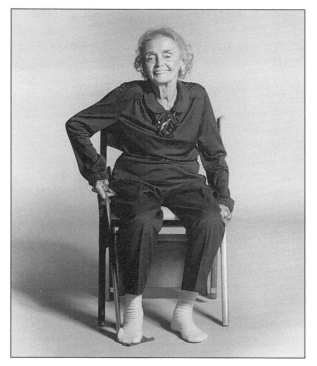

4.13 Upright row.

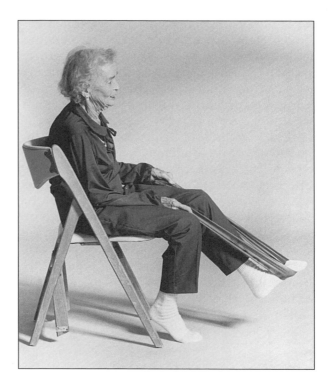

4.14 Brake push.

Keeping elbows at the sides, she pushes down with the left foot as she extends the left knee (similar to a driver stepping on the brakes), then slowly flexes the knee again to return to the starting position. The number of repetitions (from 4-12) will depend on the quadriceps and arm strength of participants. Repeat the entire sequence with the right leg. See Photo 4.14.

▋ *Knee Extension:* Exerciser ties the ends of the band into a bow (forming a circle or loop), places the loop around the right ankle, and then puts the left foot into the loop in front of the right foot (for best results, the right foot should be slightly back under the chair). Seniors should perform 4-12 left knee extensions while keeping the right leg stationary (as an anchor point). Repeat the exercise with the left leg as the anchor point and the right leg performing the knee extensions. See Photo 4.15.

COORDINATION ACTIVITIES

You can use a variety of arm movements with simple leg movements to promote coordination. For example, using the same-side (i.e., *unison*) arm and leg, exercisers touch the right foot to the front while pushing or swinging the right arm forward, then return to neutral (allow 1

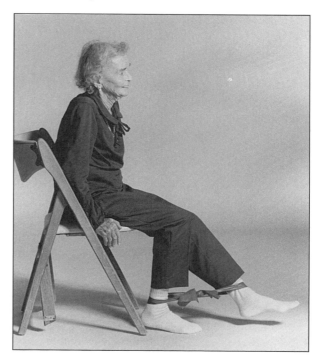

4.15 Knee extension.

count for each move). Repeat using the left foot and arm. Then they touch the right foot to the right side while pushing or swinging both arms to the right side, and return to neutral (1 count each); repeat using the left foot and both arms.

For variation, use *opposition*: Exercisers move the right foot forward while the left arm pushes or swings forward, then return both to neutral position (1 count each); then they move the left foot forward while the right arm pushes or swings forward, and return to neutral (1 count each). Next, seniors move the right foot to the right side while both arms swing to the left; return to neutral; then move the left foot to the left side while both arms swing to the right, and return to neutral (1 count each). See Photos 4.16 a and b.

Using unison and opposition movements, you can create an endless variety of arm and leg exercises that require both concentration and coordination to perform. Create short routines that your participants can learn and practice, set to music they like. Being able to complete a challenging routine gives your students a real boost in self-esteem, and it's fun!

RHYTHMICS AND FUN

Many rhythmic activities can be modified for chair exercise. You can use folk and square dance patterns by marching in place and using knee lifts instead of the normal traveling steps. For coordination rhythmics, you can develop movements to be performed in 8-count, 4-count,

and 2-count sets. For example: 8 toe touches forward, 8 heel presses forward, 8 touches to alternating sides, 8 kicks forward, 8 knee lifts; then repeat the sequence using 4 counts of each, 2 counts of each, and finally 1 count of each.

It is also fun to use imagery. Going for a "walk in the forest" could include mimicking movements such as walking up a steep incline, running from a bear, climbing a tree, or picking up pine cones. You can either make up the story yourself or ask each participant to contribute one movement for the story. Or act out a familiar rhyme, like "The Noble Duke of York," to promote quadriceps strength for maintaining the ability to easily rise from and sit down on chairs. Start in neutral position and begin marching in place reciting, "The noble Duke of York, he had 10,000 men; he marched them (up) the hill and marched them (down) again. When they were (up) they were up, and when they were (down) they were down, and when they were only halfway up, they were neither (up) nor (down)." Each time "up" occurs in parentheses, participants stand up, and each time "down" occurs in parentheses, they sit back down. At the phrase "when they were only halfway up," participants stand in a crouched position, knees slightly bent, straightening the knees

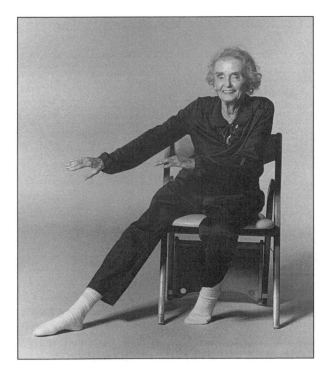

4.16a Coordination—unison.

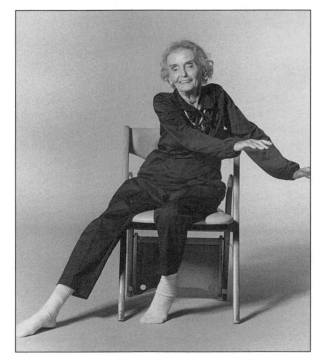

4.16b Coordination—opposition.

fully only at the next "(up)." Use your imagination to incorporate other rhymes with action words that could promote "movement that matters."

SOCIALIZATION

It is important to set aside time in your chair-exercise class for socialization. This allows (and encourages) everyone to share news about what's happening with their family, friends, or themselves. It is also an excellent time to share special thoughts for the day, short poems, or inspirational writings. When this becomes a regular part of class, your seniors will often bring things they have heard or read to share with their classmates.

THE BASIC EXERCISE CLASS

The most common target audience for a basic exercise class is the slightly impaired or restricted senior and the sedentary senior. Set goals for this class to improve range of motion, strength, coordination, and balance and to achieve low-level cardiovascular benefits. You may utilize all of the chair and chair-assisted exercises and activities described previously and also incorporate walking, station work, wall work, and standing rhythmic exercises.

Caution: A percentage of the participants in a basic exercise class will likely suffer from some level of osteoporosis. The cautions outlined in the chair exercise portion of this book also apply to this class. Avoid fully compressing the abdominal area as well as any rapid, jerky movements. Also avoid standing on one leg for more than 8 counts at a time and movements that involve twisting while standing on one leg.

WALKING COURSES AND STATIONS

Walking is an excellent exercise for seniors and one of the most popular. To add interest and fun to the walking portion of the basic exercise class, set up a walking course in the facility. Have exercise stations around the area with posters illustrating the exercises to do at each station. Each station should concentrate on one specific fitness goal, so include a wide range of exercises dealing with range of motion, strength, balance, and coordination. Some of these can include wall work, such as wall push-ups and other wall-supported activities.

You can also create an "accumulated mileage" program that records the number of miles walked in the facility and gives the participants "credit" for the miles on a charted course. For example, the class may decide that they want to "walk across America." Let 1 mile walked in class equal 100 miles (or whatever you decide is appropriate) on a "walk across America" and chart your participants' progress across a map posted in the facility. Be sure to provide incentives for reaching certain landmarks or minigoals along the way. This type of program allows unlimited opportunities for fun activities and celebrations related to the class's "travels."

WALL EXERCISES

Wall exercises are a useful supplement to exercises done in the chair or with chair support. *Front neutral* position is defined as standing facing the wall with both palms on the wall. *Right-side neutral* is standing with the left side toward the wall, the left palm on the wall, and the left elbow slightly flexed. *Left-side neutral* is standing with the right side to the wall, right palm on the wall, and right elbow slightly flexed.

■ *Push-Ups:* Exercisers stand in front neutral position approximately 12 to 15 inches away from the wall, feet together and palms flat against the wall at shoulder height and shoulder width. They lower themselves toward the wall by bending the elbows, and then push away from the wall by straightening the elbows, keeping the palms in contact with the wall, the back straight, and feet flat on the floor while executing the movements slowly. To create more resistance for improved upper body strength, this exercise may be performed with a stretchy band placed around the back, one end grasped in each hand. As the exercisers push away from the wall, they also push against the resistance of the stretchy band. See Photo 4.17.

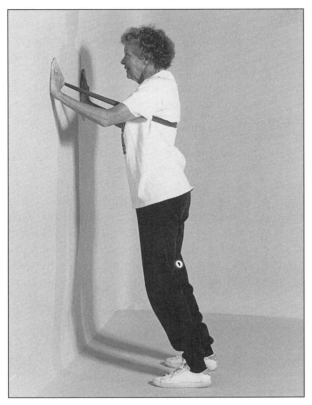

4.17 Wall push-up with resistance band.

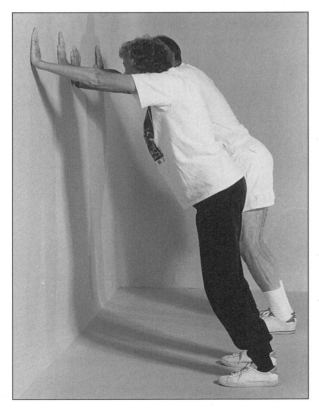

4.18 Wall crawl.

Caution: Those with joint difficulties should avoid flexing the elbow more than 90 degrees against resistance.

▌ **Wall Crawl:** This exercise begins in front neutral position, very close to the wall with the hands at shoulder level. The exerciser crawls his fingers up the wall reaching to the highest point possible, even rising on to his toes (8 counts), holds for 8 counts, then crawls fingers back down the wall (8 counts) and steps back away from the wall (hands still in contact), flattens the back and looks down between the outstretched arms (8 counts). During the sequence, the knees should be slightly flexed and the back as flat as possible. See Photo 4.18.

▌ **Shoulder Stretch:** Beginning in left-side neutral position, the exerciser turns slowly away from the wall to look over the left shoulder, and holds for 8 counts, then returns slowly to neutral position. She then repeats the movement in right-side neutral position, turning to look over the right shoulder. See Photo 4.19.

▌ **Wall Sits:** With their backs to the wall and feet approximately 12 to 15 inches away, the participants flex their knees until they are in a position similar to sitting in a chair. (Do not go past a 90-degree flexion.) Then they straighten the knees with the back still against the wall to recover. Exercisers should work up to holding this "sitting" position for about 15 seconds at a time. See Photo 4.20.

Caution: Do not allow those who are unsteady on their feet, or who have very weak quadriceps muscles, to perform wall sits.

▌ **Side Leg-Lifts:** Beginning in right-side neutral position, the exerciser does small side leg-lifts with the right leg, keeping the right toe pointing straight forward (no turnout) and the foot flexed. The supporting leg should also be slightly flexed. Exercisers should do a maximum of 8 consecutive lifts on one side before switching to the other side.

▌ **Side Stretch:** Beginning in right-side neutral, exercisers reach overhead and continue reaching over to the wall with their right

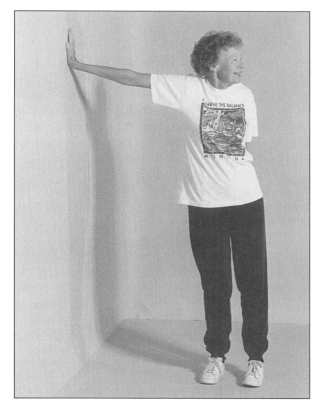

4.19 Shoulder stretch.

arm (Counts 1, 2, 3, 4), bending at the waist. They hold the stretch over Counts 5, 6, 7, 8 and 1, 2, 3, 4, then return to neutral by bringing the right arm down in front of the body (5, 6, 7, 8). Exercisers may repeat the stretch 4 times on the right side, then switch to left-side neutral position.

▌*Calf Stretch:* The participant begins in front neutral position with the right toe against the wall, the right knee flexed. While extending the left foot back in a wide lunge, keeping the left leg straight (i.e., right forward lunge position), she presses the left heel toward the floor for 8 to 12 counts. She then repeats the movement, extending the right foot back.

▌*Quad Stretch:* Beginning in right-side neutral, exercisers bring the right heel toward the buttock by flexing the right knee and grasping the right ankle with the right hand. They hold this stretch, keeping the right knee pointed straight down to the floor and the left knee slightly flexed. Caution them not to hyperextend the lower back. Repeat with the left leg.

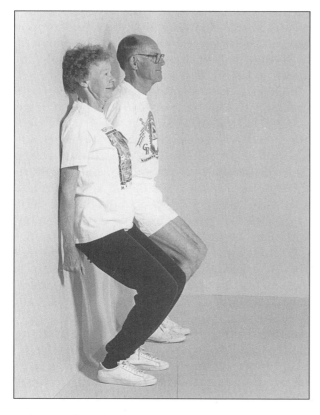

4.20 Wall sits

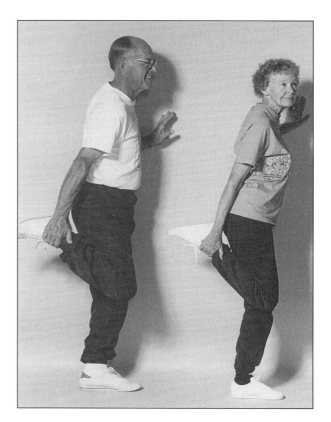

4.21 Quad stretch.

Caution: The heel should not touch the buttocks, because this hyperflexes the knee, placing it in a position vulnerable to injury. A stretchy band or old tie can be looped around the ankle to assist those who are unable to comfortably grasp their ankle. See Photo 4.21.

❚ *Balance:* Exercisers can also do balance work at the wall, raising onto the toes, holding their balance on one foot, or doing small single leg raises to the front or back. The wall provides a safe support when needed.

STANDING RHYTHMIC EXERCISES

Standing rhythmic exercise can be incorporated easily into the basic exercise class. The simple toe touches and heel presses forward, to the sides, and to the back, as well as small kicks and knee lifts described on pages 58 and 59 (Photos 4.22, 4.23 and 4.24), can safely be used with this group. However, because seniors who participate in this level of class may have some difficulty with balance, it is important that they always have support while they are performing the standing rhythmic exercises, whether chair-assisted support, standing next to a wall with one hand on the wall, or holding hands in a circle. If your participants hold hands in a circle during balance activities, be aware of participants' size and strength variations. Make sure that very small individuals are not holding hands with considerably larger people who may pull them off balance during the movements.

LOW-IMPACT AEROBICS

The target audience for this class is the healthy, active senior who has enough mobility to move easily from one foot to the other and not require assistance in walking forward, backward, or sideways. Low-impact aerobics are geared toward improving aerobic condition through continuous movement to music, with stretching and strengthening exercises mixed in. Goals include improved cardiovascular fitness, strength, flexibility, balance, and coordination.

CLASS FORMAT

A low-impact class for seniors should begin with a 10- to 20-minute warm-up of continuous easy movement to music to increase the circulation and help everyone become comfortable with moving. A 20- to 25-minute aerobic phase follows the warm-up and should include careful monitoring of exercise intensity (described in chapter 3). This phase will also include range-of-motion and strength movements.

The final phase is a 15- to 20-minute cooldown, including balance and coordination work, and then relaxation and socialization activities. This is a good time to pass along health information and words of wisdom or humor or to conduct an open forum for sharing thoughts. It is important to actually schedule class time for and to plan ways to facilitate socialization. Some will occur on its own but it is up to you as instructor to set the tone of the class by making sure that the social aspect is a priority.

SAFE MOVEMENT

The main core of the movement should stay very simple so that everyone in class is successful in movement most of the time. Complicated combinations and patterns of movement will frustrate the average senior and add an unwanted element of stress.

To keep the class interesting, utilize a large variety of arm movements. Movements that use opposing arms and legs alternated with movements that use same-side arms and legs (unison) add variety and improve coordination. For added interest, vary your exercise formation, alternating among front-facing rows, circles, lines, and partners. Many folk dances and simple line dances can also be modified for safety and incorporated into your exercise program.

While trying to add variety and interest, remember to evaluate *all* movements in terms of the benefits versus the risks. For example, movements traveling to the side should not be done until the class has spent adequate time warming up the muscles of the hips and legs by doing toe and heel touches to the sides and front. Side-to-side sliding steps and fast cross-over steps (such as grapevines) pose a high risk of falling and therefore should not be used.

When switching to new patterns of movement, marching in place is an excellent transition step and should be used between changes of direction or in the movement pattern. This allows everyone to become centered before trying to change directions or focusing on a new series of steps. Use hand signals as well as verbal cues while marching in place to indicate to the class the direction in which you intend to travel.

SPECIFIC EXERCISES

The following are descriptions and illustrations of exercise movements that can be used for the warm-up, aerobic, and cool-down phases. During the warm-up phase, exercises done to slow music concentrate on increasing circulation and working through the range of motions that participants will be using during the aerobic

Table 4.1 Low-Impact Land-Based Exercise

Leg Movements				Arm Movements			
Exercise	Warm-up	Aerobic	Cool-down	Exercise	Warm-up	Aerobic	Cool-down
Stationary				Single or double arm circles (elbows slightly bent)	√	√	
*March	√	√	√				
*Toe touch, front	√	√	√	Windshield wipers	√	√	
*Toe touch, side	√	√	√	Biceps curls	√	√	
Toe touch, back	√	√		Arm swings (opposite side as leg)	√	√	√
*Heel press, forward	√	√	√				
*Heel press, side	√	√	√	Arm swings (same side as leg)	√	√	√
*Small kicks, front	√	√					
*Knee lifts	√	√		Arm swings (1 arm fwd, 1 bkwd)	√	√	√
Knee lift, side diagonal	√	√		Arm swings (both fwd, bkwd)	√	√	√
Knee lift, small kick (chorus line)	√	√		Arm waves overhead		√	
Heel lifts to back	√		√	Palm press, overhead	√	√	
Toe touch, fwd, side, bk, step	√		√	Palm press, forward	√	√	√
				Palm press, side	√	√	√
Toe touch, fwd, side, fwd, step	√		√	Palm press, down	√	√	√
Charleston	√	√		Palm press, diagonal overhead	√	√	
Modified box step	√	√		Arm crosses	√	√	
Side step touch	√	√	√	Front and back crawl	√	√	
				Scarecrow	√	√	
Traveling							
Exercises above marked by asterisk	√	√	√				
Step, touch (moving fwd or bk)	√	√	√	**Transitions: Helpful Hints**			
Two-step	√	√		• Always start with one part moving first then add a second part later. Example: Start moving the feet first, then add an arm movement.			
Hustle step, forward	√	√					
Hustle step, side	√	√		• Return to center (marching) before changing directions of movement.			
Walk or march fwd; bkwd; own circle; large circle holding hands	√	√	√	• When in a circle, give the command "Look R" (or L), "Turn R" (or L), "Move R" (or L), etc., so everyone knows which direction to move.			

phase. Movement is faster and more vigorous done to upbeat music during the aerobic phase, when you concentrate on elevating the heart rate to the training zone. During the cool-down phase, movements are slow again to bring the heart rate down gradually and prepare the body for stretching. Table 4.1 outlines exercises that can be used in any phase and those that are exclusive to a particular phase.

Neutral position is defined as facing forward, standing with weight equally distributed on both feet, and having arms relaxed at the sides. While performing any exercise movement, seniors should keep the knees slightly flexed to promote better balance and to ease the transfer of weight from one foot to the other.

Stationary Movements

▌ *Marching in Place:* A simple march step (left foot, right foot, left, right, etc.) is an excellent transitional movement to use immediately before changing directions of travel and to return to often. From 8 to 24 counts of marching is appropriate for a transition step.

▌ *Heel Presses:* With the weight on the left foot, the exerciser extends the right foot out, pressing the heel to the front (Count 1), and brings the right foot back to neutral stepping on the right foot (2). Then she extends the left foot out, pressing the heel to the front (3), and brings the left foot back to neutral and steps on the left foot (4). Repeat the movement: right-heel press, step, left-heel press, step, etc.

Heel presses can also be done to the sides. The participant extends the right foot to the right side diagonal (Count 1), brings the foot back to neutral and steps on right foot (2), then extends the left foot to the left side diagonal (3), brings it back to neutral and steps on left foot (4), etc. Heel presses should not be done touching back.

▌ *Toe Touches:* Participants perform the sequence of movement described in the heel presses but, instead of pressing with the heel, they touch the toe out—forward for front toe touch, directly to the side for side toe touches. Toe touches can be performed to the back, as shown in Photo 4.23.

▌ *Small Kicks:* Participants perform the sequence of movement described in the heel presses except, instead of pressing with the heel, they give a small kick with the foot and lower leg well below the knee. Small kicks can be performed to the front or to the side diagonal but should *not* be attempted to the back

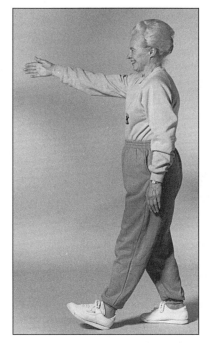

4.22 Heel presses.

4.23 Toe touches.

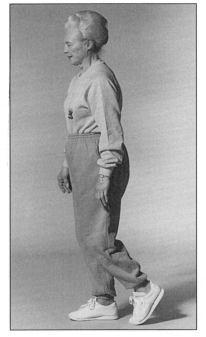

4.24 Small kicks.

█ *Knee Lifts:* With the weight on the left foot, the senior exerciser lifts the right knee up (Count 1), steps onto the right foot next to the left foot (2), lifts the left knee up (3), steps onto the left foot next to the right foot (4), repeating for a set number of reps. Knee lifts can be performed to the front or to the diagonal side. They can also be performed as doubles; that is, lift right knee (Count 1), touch right foot to floor (2), lift right knee again (3), then step on the right foot (4). Do not ask participants to perform knee lifts directly to the side; this requires an advanced degree of hip rotation, which is unsafe for many seniors while standing on one leg.

█ *Chorus Line* (Knee lift, small kick): With the weight on the left foot, the participant lifts the right knee (Count 1), touches the right toe to the floor next to the left foot (2), gives a small kick with the right foot and lower leg (3), and steps on the right foot (4), then repeats the sequence with the left leg.

█ *Heel Lifts Back:* With the weight on the left foot, exercisers bend the right knee and lift the right heel toward the buttock on Count 1 (the knee should flex approximately 90 degrees), step on the right foot (2), lift the left heel toward the buttock (3), and then step on the left foot (4). They should perform this movement with a controlled bending of the knee rather than flinging the heel toward the buttock.

█ *Toe Touches Front, Side, Back, and Step:* With the weight on the left foot, the exerciser touches the right toe to the front (Count 1), then to the right side (2), to the back (3), and then steps on the right foot next to the left foot (4). He then repeats the sequence with the left foot—touch left foot front (5), to the left (6), to the back (7)—and finally steps on the left foot (8). A simple variation of this movement has the exerciser touching front, side, front again, and step.

█ *Charleston:* With the weight on the left foot, the participant gives a small kick forward with the right foot (Count 1), steps on the right foot next to the left (2), touches the left foot to the back (3), then steps on the left foot next to the right foot (4). Continue this sequence for a number of reps. To perform the exercise on the left side, the participant starts with the weight on the right foot and begins the sequence by kicking forward with the left foot.

█ *Box Step:* With the weight on the left foot, the exerciser steps forward onto the right foot (Count 1), forward onto the left foot (2), back onto the right foot (3), and then back onto the left foot (4).

█ *Side Step, Touch:* With the weight on the left foot, participants step to the right side onto the right foot (Count 1), touch the left toe next to the right foot (2), step to the left side onto the left foot (3), then touch the right toe next to the left foot (4). See Photos 4.25 a and b.

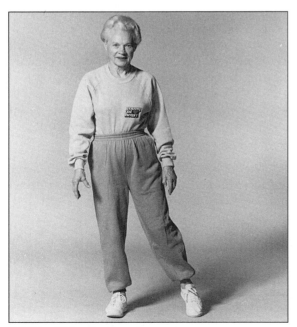

4.25a Side-step touch.

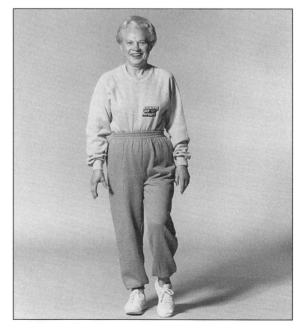

4.25b Side-step touch.

Traveling Movements

∎ *Marching:*   Progress forward or backward with each step.

∎ *Toe Touches, Heel Presses, and Small Kicks:*   Instead of returning the foot to neutral after doing the toe touch, heel press, or small kick (Counts 1, 3, 5, 7), have participants step forward or backward on Counts 2, 4, 6, and 8. Toe touches to the back should *not* travel nor should small kicks to the side diagonal.

∎ *Knee Lifts:*   Instead of stepping down next to the weight-bearing foot after the knee lift (Counts 1, 3, 5, 7), exercisers step forward or backward on Counts 2, 4, 6, and 8. Double knee lifts should *not* travel.

∎ *Step Touch:*   With the weight on the left foot, exercisers step forward onto the right foot (Count 1), touch the left toe next to the right foot (2), then step forward onto the left foot (3), and touch the right toe next to the left foot (4). This movement can progress backward by having exercisers step backward onto the foot (Counts 1 and 3) instead of forward.

∎ *Two-Step:*   With the weight on the left foot, participants step forward onto the right foot (Count 1), then onto the left foot closing next to the right foot (&), step forward onto the right foot (2); step forward onto the left foot past the right foot (3), step onto the right foot closing next to the left foot (&), step forward onto the left foot (4). The cueing phrase is "forward right, close, right; forward left, close, left."

∎ *Hustle Step:*   Beginning with the weight on the left foot, exercisers travel forward stepping right (Count 1), left (2), right (3), and touch the left toe next to the right foot (4). They repeat the movement but travel backward by stepping *back* onto the left foot (5), right foot (6), left foot (7), and touch the right toe next to the left foot (8). The cueing phrase is "forward right, left, right, tap left; backward left, right, left, tap right."

∎ *Hustle Step Side:*   With the weight on the left foot, exercisers step right onto the right foot (Count 1), bring the left foot next to the right foot and step onto the left foot (2), step to the right side again onto the right foot (3), then touch the left toe next to your right foot (4).

They repeat the sequence but travel to the left by stepping left (5), close right next to left (6), step to left (7), and touch with the right toe (8). The cueing phrase is "side right, close, right, tap left; side left, close, left, tap right."

Arm Movements

Always start one body part moving before adding a second. For example, start with a foot movement and, when you can see that all class members are doing it correctly, add an arm movement. The neutral position is arms hanging down in a relaxed position next to the sides of the body.

∎ *Arm Circles:*   Exercisers circle one or both arms to the front, or out to the sides, keeping the elbow(s) slightly bent throughout the motion.

∎ *Windshield Wipers:*   With both arms in front of the body, elbows flexed, palms turned forward, participants sweep both arms to the right and then to the left, mimicking the action of windshield wipers.

∎ *Biceps Curls:*   Exercisers extend both arms down in front of the body with palms facing up. They flex the right elbow (palm up), then while straightening the right elbow, flex the left elbow (palm up). Repeat the motion with the cues, "Flex right, left, right, left." Curls may also be done with light 1- to 3-pound weights.

∎ *Arm Swings:*   The participant swings one or both arms to the side, forward, or backward. Arm swings can be done in opposition to the leg work or in unison (i.e., same-side leg and arm). They can also be done one arm swinging forward while the other arm swings back, either in opposition or in unison with the leg work. Allow 2 counts for each swing in any direction. See Photos 4.26a and b.

∎ *Arm Waves Overhead:*   With the arms extended over the head, palms facing out, participants sway both arms right, left, right, left. This can also be done with one arm extended overhead.

∎ *Palm Presses:*   Beginning in neutral position, exercisers flex one or both elbows bringing the hands toward the shoulders, then extend the elbows by pressing out with the wrists flexed and palms turned straight up (palm press up), to the front (palm press forward), to the sides (palm press side), or straight down (palm press down). This can also be done with one arm at a time pressing up, forward, side, down, or at a diagonal, crossing overhead. See Photo 4.27.

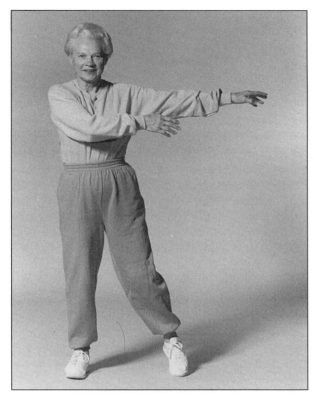

4.26a Arm swings unison.

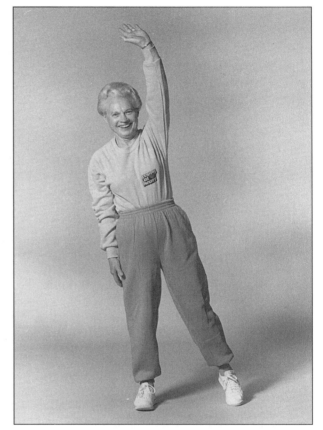

4.27 Palm press diagonal.

❚ Arm Crosses: Beginning in neutral position, participants lift and cross both arms in front of the body (1 count for each movement) right over left, and open to sides; then cross both arms behind the body left over right, and open to sides. These can be done at hip level. Front arm crosses can also be done at chest level, alternating right over left, then left over right. The elbows should be slightly bent.

❚ Front and Back Crawls: With the elbows flexed, participants mimic the action of a front or back stroke in swimming. When performing the back crawl, they should allow the elbows to lead the stroke (allow 2-4 counts each stroke).

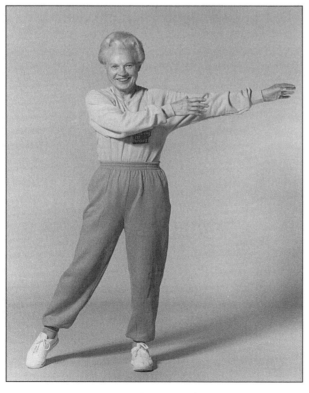

4.26b Opposition

■ **Scarecrow:**   Beginning in neutral position, exercisers lift the bent elbows out to the sides, forearms perpendicular to the floor, palms facing backward, then straighten the arms to the sides by extending the elbows while keeping the palms facing backward. They continue the movement, flexing and extending the elbows.

Wall Exercises

Wall exercises can be used in place of or in conjunction with floor exercises to promote strength and flexibility. Some seniors are uncomfortable doing floor exercises and prefer working against the wall. All of the wall exercises described for a basic exercise class can be used in the cool-down phase of a low-impact aerobics class. (See pages 53-56 for complete descriptions of these exercises.)

Floor Exercises

Floor exercises should always be done on a mat or other soft surface. If your facility does not provide large mats, there are many different kinds of affordable individual exercise mats that your class members may purchase. If you have a senior who is unable or unwilling to use the mat, you can modify some exercises to be done in a chair or against the wall.

■ **Curl-Ups:**   Lying in neutral back position (i.e., on the back, feet flat on the floor, knees flexed) with hands either behind the neck (not on the head) or crossed in front of the chest, the exerciser performs slow, small curl-ups with the shoulders no more than 6 inches off the floor. Seniors should do no more than 10 repetitions at a time to avoid stress on the neck. Alternate curl-ups with hamstring stretches, hip tucks, or other floor work that puts the neck in a totally relaxed position.

■ **Knee Hug:**   Beginning in neutral back position, participants wrap the arms under the knees and bring the knees slowly to the chest, holding to gently stretch the lower back, while breathing normally. Hold for 12 to 16 counts.

■ **Hamstring Stretch:**   From neutral back position, exercisers extend the right knee so that the right leg points straight up with the foot flexed and hold the leg in this position to stretch the right hamstring. A stretch band, an old tie, or any strip of fabric can be used to assist in this stretch. Wrap the aid around the sole of the foot and use it to help keep the leg in a stretched position. Repeat the stretch on the left side. See Photo 4.28

■ **Frog Sit:**   Participants sit with knees out to the sides and the soles of the feet together. They place the elbows on the knees and gently push down to stretch the muscles of the inner thighs. See Photo 4.29.

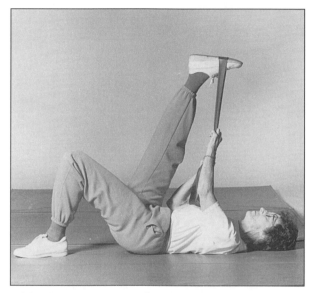

4.28   Hamstring stretch.

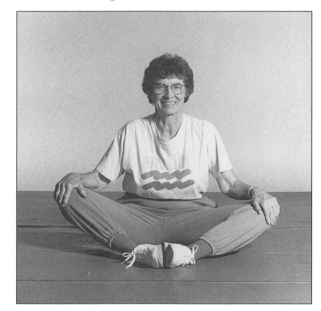

4.29   Frog sit.

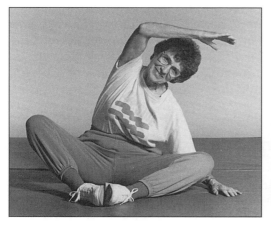

4.30 Frog sit with side reach.

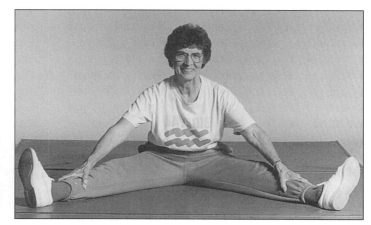

4.31 Saddle stretch.

■ *Frog Sit With Side Reach:* Beginning in frog-sit position, exercisers place the left hand on the floor next to the left leg and gently drop over to the left side, stretching the muscles on the right side of the body. Then they repeat the stretch to the right side. A more advanced stretch is to reach the arm up and over the head to the side.

■ *Straddle Stretch:* Participants sit straight up with their legs extended open to the sides. Keeping the back and the legs straight, they slowly flex forward at the hips until they feel a stretch in the hamstring and hip extensor muscles. Hold the stretch for 8 to 16 counts. Some people will feel a stretch just by getting into the beginning position trying to keep the back and the legs straight.

■ *Lower Back Stretch:* Lying on their backs with the legs extended straight out on the mat, exercisers bend the right knee and place the right foot next to the left knee, then gently allow the right knee to cross over the top of the left leg while trying to keep both shoulders on the floor. Hold the stretch for 12 to 24 counts, reminding participants to breathe normally. Return to neutral, then repeat the stretch to the left side.

■ *Side Leg Lift:* Lying on the left side with the hips in a line perpendicular to the floor, feet pointing forward (i.e., no turnout at hip) and the ankles flexed, exercisers do small right leg lifts (8-16 reps). Not propping the head up with the left hand, they keep the left arm extended flat onto the mat with the head resting on the left arm. Then they repeat the exercise lying on the right side.

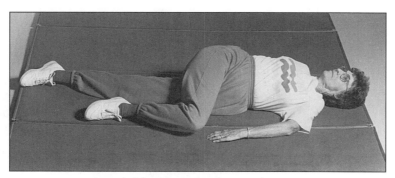

4.32 Lower back stretch.

▌ *Modified Push-Up:* Participants begin by lying face down on the mat with both palms flat on the mat next to the shoulders. Slowly, they raise the body from the mat by pushing with the hands and extending the elbows while keeping the legs from the knees down on the mat. With the back straight and the head in line with the neck and back, they lower themselves down until the chest almost touches the mat and then push up again, fully extending the elbows. If some of your participants lack the strength to do the push-up, have them begin in an elbows-extended position and lower themselves to the mat.

▌ *Hip Tuck:* Lying in the neutral back position, exercisers tuck the hips upward by contracting the lower abdominal muscles and buttocks. They hold this position for 4 to 8 counts, then return to the neutral back position. This is a very small movement during which participants should keep most of the back in contact with the floor.

▌ *Cat Arch:* Beginning with hands and knees on the mat, participants arch their backs (like an angry cat), hold, and then release to the beginning position. Remind them to breathe normally.

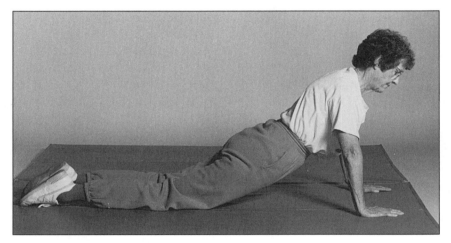

4.33 Modified push-up.

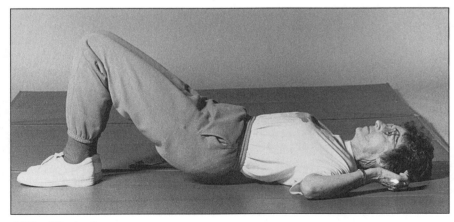

4.34 Hip tuck.

▌ *Low Back Strength:* Exercisers lie face down on the mat with the elbows and lower arms flat, palms down. They slowly raise the upper body off the mat about 6 to 8 inches and hold (4 to 8 counts), then return to beginning position. See Photo 4.35. Seniors should not push with the arms; the back should do the work, the arms providing balance and support, if needed.

Balance and Coordination

For balance activities, have the seniors stand either next to a wall or in the center of the floor in lines or in a circle holding hands. Use balance activities during the cool-down *only*.

▌ *Leg Lift:* Exercisers do small straight-leg lifts (approximately 6 inches off the floor) to the front or to the front diagonal. Hold for a maximum of 12 counts before changing to the other leg.

▌ *Knee Lift:* Participants lift one knee to the front at a 90-degree angle, and hold for a maximum of 12 counts.

▌ *Knee Lift With Cross:* With the weight on the left leg, exercisers lift the right knee to center (Count 1), cross the right leg over the left leg and touch the right toe to the left of the left foot (2), lift the right knee back to center (3), and then step onto the right foot (4). They repeat the movement crossing left leg over right. See Photos 4.36 a and b.

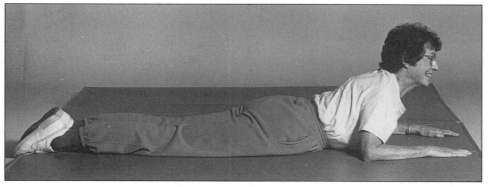

4.35 Low back strength.

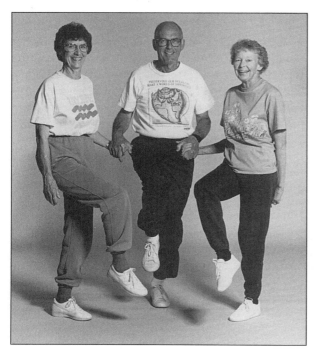

4.36a Knee lift cross.

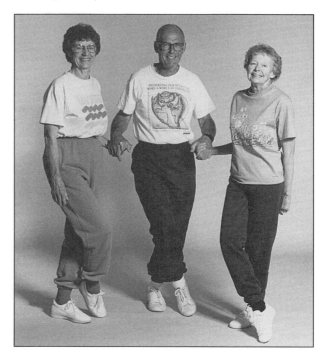

4.36b Knee lift cross.

■ *Relevé:* Standing next to a wall, or in lines or circles holding hands, participants raise up onto the toes and balance for 8 counts, then return the heels to the floor and bend the knees (keeping the heels on the floor). They repeat the relevé sequence 4 to 8 times.

■ *Toe Tap:* Standing in a circle holding hands, exercisers extend the right leg to the front and tap the right toe, using the ankle to flex and tap the toe. They tap 1, 2, 3, 4, 5, 6, 7, step onto the right foot (8), then repeat with the left foot tapping 7 counts, then step onto the left foot (8). You may repeat the sequence using a countdown of 4, then 2 on each foot.

■ *Side Steps:* Standing in a circle holding hands, exercisers step to the right onto the right foot (1), step the left foot next to the right (2), step to the right on the right foot (3), tap with the left foot beside the right foot (4). They repeat the sequence, traveling to the left (5, 6, 7, 8), ending with a tap with the right foot. Step to the right with the right foot (1), tap with the left foot beside the right foot (2), step to the left with the left foot (3), tap with the right foot beside the left foot (4), and repeat the movement to the right, tap, left, tap, for Counts 5, 6, 7, and 8. Cue the sequence, "Step right, close, right, tap left; step left, close, left, tap right; step right, tap, step left, tap, step right, tap, step left, tap."

Social Interaction

Use a variety of formations to help facilitate social interaction throughout the entire class period. For example, a large circle with participants holding hands for parts of the warm-up, aerobic, and cool-down allows everyone to see each other, exchange smiles, and even talk a little (especially good for the cool-down phase). Two lines that face each other also allow exchanges between class members and make a

good transition to partner work. You can also develop activities that are specifically designed to foster interaction.

■ *Shoulder Rub:* Have the participants find partners who are approximately their same height. Have one of the partners stand behind the other and give him or her a shoulder rubdown, then switch places. This can also be done in a small circle.

■ *Writing Names:* With partners, one person stands behind the other and writes the other's name on her or his back; then they switch places. This feels great and is also a good way to help participants learn and remember each other's names.

■ *Ball Toss:* Have participants form a circle. Begin by calling out your own name and handing a ball to the person next to you. The rest of the people in the circle repeat your name in unison. The ball continues around the circle as each person calls out his or her name, all participants in unison repeat the name, and the person passes the ball to the next person.

After one time around the circle, the last person holding the ball calls out a name and tosses the ball to that person. This is a fun activity that helps people remember names and exercises eye-hand coordination. Either a large rubber ball or a small Kooshie ball is a good choice for this activity.

■ *Sharing Time:* Set aside some time in class each week to be a sharing time when people can bring in a thought for the day, a poem, a funny anecdote, health tips, or just share something that is happening in their lives. Have several items prepared to share with the class in case others do not bring anything. When this becomes a regular part of your class, people will bring items to share with others more frequently.

CHAPTER

5

Water-Based Programming

Water-exercise programs enjoy wide appeal. The target audiences for these classes may include healthy but sedentary seniors or seniors recovering from an injury or surgery. Many seniors are referred to water exercise by their physicians to aid recovery from hip, knee, or back surgery. But healthy, active seniors also enjoy the water and the type of vigorous but gentle workout it can provide. So, if possible offer a variety of levels of water exercise to meet the needs of this range of functional abilities.

This chapter addresses special concerns you must evaluate when developing senior water-exercise classes, and gives specific programming for water aerobics, Levels 1 and 2, and for arthritis water exercise.

SPECIAL CONSIDERATIONS

You must pay close attention to a number of special considerations to ensure that your water-exercise program can safely meet the needs of the older adult population. These considerations include knowing target heart rate variations appropriate to water exercise, the special safety aspects unique to a pool environment, and a pool temperature that allows for the comfort of your senior participants when in the wa-

ter. They also involve special musical needs warranted by the generally poor acoustics in a pool area and the likelihood of having to deal with uncorrected hearing impairments.

TARGET HEART RATE VARIATIONS

It is critical that you and your participants be aware that the target heart rate zones for water exercise are different than those for land exercise. There are conflicting theories as to why the significant difference, but the generally accepted adjustment factor is -17 beats per minute. (Figure 5.1 illustrates the Karvonen formula modified for senior water exercise). Form a habit of requiring your students to call out their 10-second exercise pulse rates whenever you point to them during the heart rate check. In addition to the target heart rate, all participants should use their rates of perceived exertion (explained in chapter 3 and illustrated in Figure 3.3, p. 33) to monitor exercise intensity. When you ask your participants to take their pulse rate or judge their levels of exertion, use clear, easy-to-follow commands each time, being sensitive to the fact that many of them will not be wearing their glasses or hearing aids while in the water.

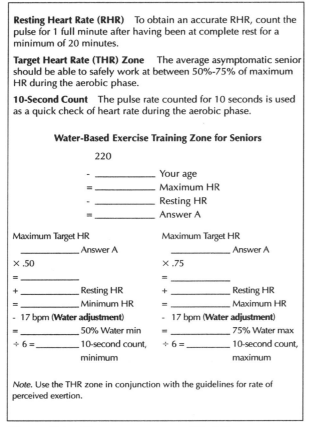

Resting Heart Rate (RHR)　To obtain an accurate RHR, count the pulse for 1 full minute after having been at complete rest for a minimum of 20 minutes.

Target Heart Rate (THR) Zone　The average asymptomatic senior should be able to safely work at between 50%-75% of maximum HR during the aerobic phase.

10-Second Count　The pulse rate counted for 10 seconds is used as a quick check of heart rate during the aerobic phase.

Water-Based Exercise Training Zone for Seniors

220

- _____ Your age
= _____ Maximum HR
- _____ Resting HR
= _____ Answer A

Maximum Target HR	Maximum Target HR
_____ Answer A	_____ Answer A
× .50	× .75
= _____	= _____
+ _____ Resting HR	+ _____ Resting HR
= _____ Minimum HR	= _____ Maximum HR
- 17 bpm (**Water adjustment**)	- 17 bpm (**Water adjustment**)
= _____ 50% Water min	= _____ 75% Water max
÷ 6 = _____ 10-second count, minimum	÷ 6 = _____ 10-second count, maximum

Note. Use the THR zone in conjunction with the guidelines for rate of perceived exertion.

Figure 5.1　Water-exercise modified Karvonen formula.

SAFETY

Safety is always the highest priority in a senior exercise class. The special conditions imposed by the pool environment present some additional safety concerns that you must address in your water-exercise program. For example, in addition to the CPR and first aid qualifications required of a senior-exercise instructor, a water-exercise instructor may need to have training in emergency water safety. If there is a lifeguard on duty during the water-exercise class, you may not be required to have emergency water safety training. However, if you alone will be responsible for the complete safety of the participants in the pool area, you must have lifeguard certification.

Poolside Versus In-Pool Teaching

When you have the responsibility of lifeguard as well as teacher, you should teach while standing on the pool deck. It is impossible to effectively monitor both the exercise participants and the entire pool area while in the water. Besides, in a senior water-exercise class, several other factors make it more advantageous for the instructor to teach on the poolside.

First, the diminished levels of vision and hearing common to a senior population make it very difficult for participants to hear and clearly see an instructor who is teaching from the water. Second, it is much easier for class members to follow exercises that are being clearly demonstrated on the deck. Finally, and most importantly, when teaching from the deck, *you* can clearly see each of the participants. This allows you to tell if someone is performing an exercise incorrectly. It also provides you with continuous feedback from facial expressions, which means you are immediately aware if someone is having difficulty with the exercise intensity.

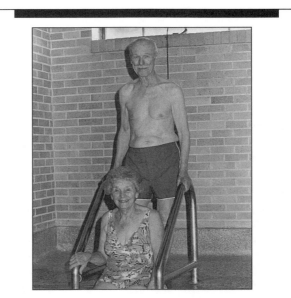

Bill and Mary Walters have been taking the senior water-exercise class 2 to 3 times a week for the past 9 years. Asked what motivates them to keep coming on a regular basis, Mary replies, "It starts the day out right for me. I really miss it if we are gone."

"It makes me feel much better physically and mentally," Bill adds. Mary agrees and adds that it gives her a better outlook on life. "I'm glad Bill and I are committed to exercising together." Both Bill and Mary agree that water-exercise class helps them stay healthy together—a high priority for them.

Being able to monitor continuously each person's response to the exercises is critical to maintaining the safety of a senior exercise class.

Pool Area

As a water-exercise instructor, you must consider the safety of your class participants from the moment they step into the pool area until they leave the facility. Evaluate the shower areas and pool deck for hazards such as slick spots or obstacles. If the shower or deck area is slick, ask students to wear aqua shoes or some other type of nonskid shoe. Monitor the condition of ladders and stairs into the pool, and take the appropriate measures to remedy the situation if they become slick or unstable in some way. In addition, monitor the condition of the bottom of the pool to ensure that it is free of debris and does not pose any safety hazards.

Safe Movement

Exercising in the water provides a low-impact workout, but *you* must still take care to prevent injury to your participants. To ensure an injury-free class, avoid rapid twisting and excessive jumping. Alternate the higher-impact jumping movements with movements that keep one foot on the pool bottom. Avoid jerky, out-of-the-water arm movements, which could cause shoulder soreness in seniors. Avoid performing an excessive amount of wall exercises that require students to support their body weight with their hands, arms, and shoulders.

Just as in a land-based exercise program, weigh the risks against the benefits for each movement. Ask your participants which exercises they enjoy doing and which exercises are uncomfortable for them. Ask them if they feel they are achieving the desired results and if they are experiencing any soreness after exercise. Continuous feedback from your senior students is essential if you are to tailor the class to meet their needs.

POOL TEMPERATURE

The temperature of the pool can have a significant impact on the success of a senior water-exercise program. If the water temperature is below 86 degrees Fahrenheit, it will be uncomfortable for many seniors who suffer symptoms of arthritis or muscle and joint dysfunction. Generally, a good pool temperature for senior water-exercise classes is from 87 to 88 degrees. This temperature allows for comfort during the warm-up and cool-down phases but is not so warm that it might pose a safety hazard during the aerobic phase.

Finding a pool that offers a comfortable temperature is a challenge, because many pools cater to lap swimmers who prefer a temperature ranging from 82 to 85 degrees. If the only available pool is close to 82 degrees, you will probably be unable to develop a successful senior water-exercise program. If the water temperature is closer to 85 degrees, then you may be able to adjust the structure of the class to work better at that temperature. For example, you can program more vigorous warm-up exercises to promote raising the body temperature, such as water-walking forward, sideways, and backward, flutter kicks on the side of the pool or with jugs, and bicycling with jugs. You may also utilize bicycling with jugs during strength work to keep the body temperature elevated during that phase.

After the aerobic phase, you may either shorten the cool-down and stretching phase or conduct the stretching session on the deck of the pool. If you choose to leave the pool for the stretch session, be sure the air temperature is warm and the pool deck is safe. (Stretches done against the wall are safest; see chapter 4 for descriptions and illustrations of wall exercises.) Shortening the cool-down and stretching phase, or getting out of the pool for stretching, is a compromise, but it is better than trying to stretch and relax in cold water, which causes a too rapid drop in body temperature and creates excessive discomfort for your participants.

MUSIC

Music plays an essential role in seniors' enjoyment of the class. Be aware of the poor acoustics that exist in most pool areas, and make the necessary adjustments in the volume and variety of music. The guidelines in chapter 3 on choosing music also apply to music for water exercise. The best choices for water exercise are simple, clear instrumentals with a strong, easy-to-follow beat. Simple vocals can also be used, but poor acoustics and splashing water will compete with the music and its vocal accompaniment. If you use vocals, alternate them with instrumental arrangements to provide a soothing balance of music.

General Class Format

Senior water-exercise classes begin with a warm-up that involves gentle range-of-motion activities designed to promote circulation and help the participants become comfortable with movement. Classes also include an aerobic phase that lasts from 15 to 25 minutes, depending on the participants' level of ability. These phases must include careful monitoring of the exercise intensity; check pulse rates after the warm-up exercises and again at least twice during the aerobic phase. Remember to take the exercise pulse rate immediately after the conclusion of the aerobic phase, and then 1 minute later take the recovery pulse rate. Use the target heart rate variation described in Figure 5.1. (Specific strategies for monitoring exercise intensity are presented in chapter 3.)

Include coordination movements in the warm-up and aerobic phases, varying arm movements with opposition, same-side (unison), and sequential motions. This will keep the exercise interesting while developing and improving coordination skills.

Also, remind your seniors not to stay on the balls of their feet throughout the class but instead to keep the heels in contact with the pool floor. Staying on the balls of the feet throughout the class period will seriously overwork the gastrocnemius muscle, causing soreness and possible injury.

A cool-down and stretching phase should follow the aerobics and should involve all major muscle groups. Several minutes of water walking is a good way to make sure everyone's heart rate returns to an acceptable level. Pay close attention to the gastrocnemius muscles, the lower back, and the hamstring; participants will have been working these muscles repeatedly during the aerobic phase. Utilize both the pool wall and the center of the pool for stretching exercises. Use slow, gentle stretches with no sharp movements, and develop smooth stretching sequences that promote relaxation as well as flexibility.

Level 1 Format

A Level 1 class consists of approximately 20 to 25 minutes of warm-up, range-of-motion, and strength work. It should also have 15 to 20 minutes of aerobics and 20 to 25 minutes of cool-down, stretching, and relaxation work. Use transition movements such as jogging and sculling side to side between high- and medium-intensity aerobic movements. Spend an equal amount of time in the transition movements and in the higher intensity movements. For example, have participants perform 16 to 24 knee lifts (medium intensity), followed by jogging in place for 16 to 24 counts (transition), then 16 to 24 cross-country-skiers (high intensity), followed by sculling side to side for 16 to 24 counts (transition). As they become more fit, have participants perform a higher number of the medium or high intensity movements (e.g., 24), followed by a lower number of the transition movements (e.g., 16). Another approach is to spend 30 to 40 seconds doing a medium- or high-intensity movement followed by 30 to 40 seconds of a transition movement. As the participants become more physically fit, have them perform the transition movements for a shorter duration (e.g., 30 seconds) than the medium- or high-intensity movements (e.g., 40 seconds).

Level 2 Format

A Level 2 water aerobics class consists of approximately 15 to 20 minutes of warm-up, range-of-motion, and strength work. It should also include 20 to 25 minutes of aerobics and 15 to 20 minutes of cool-down, stretch, and relaxation movements. You may use transition movements between medium- and high-intensity exercises, but spend more time in the high- and medium-intensity aerobic movements. For example, have participants do 24 to 32 knee lifts (medium intensity), followed by jogging in place for 16 to 20 counts (transition); then do 24 to 32 cross-country skiers (high intensity), followed by sculling side to side for 16 to 20 counts (transition). In the Level 2 class, you may also perform low- and medium-intensity exercises consecutively *without* a transition exercise. For example, have exercisers do 16 to 24 knee lifts (medium intensity), 16 to 24 large kicks front (medium intensity), followed by 16 to 20 counts of jogging in place (transition).

However, do *not* ask your seniors to perform two high-intensity exercises consecutively without doing a transition movement between them.

Using the timed approach, have Level 2 participants spend 40 to 50 seconds doing a medium- or high-intensity exercise followed by 20 to 30 seconds of a transition exercise. As participants become more physically fit, have them perform the medium- and high-intensity exercises for a longer duration (50 seconds) than the transition exercise (20 seconds), or perform low- and medium-intensity exercises consecutively without a transition exercise. When performing consecutive exercises, limit the combined time spent in low- and medium-intensity movements to approximately 80 seconds before returning to a transition exercise. For example, spend 30 to 40 seconds doing knee lifts (medium intensity) and 30 to 40 seconds doing large kicks (medium intensity), followed by 20 to 30 seconds doing a transition exercise.

SPECIFIC WATER EXERCISES

The specific exercises that follow can be used in both the Level 1 and Level 2 water-exercise classes. The warm-up can be very similar for both levels but, for the Level 1 class, you should program fewer repetitions of strength, wall, and jug exercises (i.e., exercises performed with empty gallon milk jugs for flotation). You can control the aerobic level by striking a balance between the transition movements and the higher intensity aerobic movements. The warm-up and cool-down phases of the class also provide a time for socializing, gaining health tips, and sharing bits of wisdom or humor. Also, devote a few minutes at the end of each class to total relaxation. Allow your participants to float in the water and relax with the lights turned down and nice, quiet music for atmosphere.

WARM-UP

The warm-up phase will include warm-up, range-of-motion, and strength exercises designed to promote circulation and prepare the body for more vigorous movement. Start working from the head down and move each joint through the range of motion you will be using during the aerobic phase of the program. Do not attempt to increase flexibility during this phase, but only move through the comfortable range of motion for each muscle and joint. Part of the warm-up can include jug exercises working on strength and range of motion.

Center Pool Warm-Ups

■ *Water-Walking:* Have students walk back and forth across the pool, using long strides and the proper foot strike pattern of heel then ball of the foot (no flat-footed steps). Water-walking may also be done moving either backward (with a foot strike of ball then heel) or sideways (stepping directly to the side). For variety, have students walk forward or backward crossing the right foot in front of the left, and then the left foot in front of the right.

■ *Power Water-Walking:* Have exercisers walk back and forth across the pool with knees bent, flat footed, taking small steps. This can be done forward, backward, sideways, or crossing the right foot in front of the left, then the left foot in front of the right.

■ *Small Prances:* Using a foot placement of toe-ball-heel to articulate the foot and ankle, exercisers prance in place or while moving across the pool.

■ *Bicycling:* Bicycling forward or backward with flotation jugs tucked under the arms is a good warm-up for the whole lower body.

■ *Flutter Kicks:* With kickboards or flotation jugs held out in front of the body, participants do flutter kicks and move themselves across the pool.

■ *Neck Range-of-Motion Exercise:* Any of the neck exercises outlined in chapter 4 can be used in a water-exercise warm-up. Choose two or three to begin your class. Alternate neck exercises with shoulder exercises to avoid fatiguing the neck muscles.

■ *Shoulder Movement:* Any of the shoulder exercises outlined in chapter 4 may be used in a water-exercise warm-up. Choose two or three exercises for this phase of your class. For variety, add knee bends to the shoulder exercises (keep the feet flat on the pool bottom).

▌ Arm Swings: Participants swing one or both arms through the water in unison or opposition forward and backward; they may also swing the arm(s) across the front or back of the body.

▌ Torso Movement: The torso isolations, contraction, and rotation exercises described in chapter 4 also work very well in the water-exercise warm-up. When performing contraction exercises, participants should bend both knees while contracting and then straighten the knees while opening the arms to the sides. When doing rotation exercises, bend the knees during the rotation to the side and straighten when returning to neutral. Keep movements slow and controlled.

▌ Hip Circles: Exercisers begin by gently pushing the hips from side to side, then draw circles with the hips, clockwise and counterclockwise.

▌ Toe-Drawing: Pulling their toes along the pool floor, participants draw circles, squares, or any shape, or write their names, addresses, phone numbers, and so on, using the foot only. For a variation, participants may write much bigger by using the whole leg as the writing instrument, moving the knee and hip joints, too.

▌ Single Leg Swings: With the weight on the left foot, exercisers swing the right leg forward and back (8 times) using the full range of motion at the hip while keeping the back straight, then repeat the movement with the weight on the right foot and swinging the left leg. This exercise can also be done by opening and closing either leg to the side or crossing one leg in front or behind the other. (Jugs or the wall can be used for balance, when necessary.)

▌ Ankle Circles: Exercisers bring the right knee to the chest and do right ankle circles (8 counts), then extend the leg (4 counts), hold (4 counts), point and flex the foot for 8 to 16 counts (2 counts each), then bend the knee back to the chest and repeat the sequence, beginning with the ankle circles. Then they switch to the opposite leg and begin by drawing the left knee to the chest.

▌ Knee Extensions: Participants bring the right knee to the chest (2 counts), extend the knee (2 counts), flex the knee (2 counts), then repeat extensions and flexions for 8 to 12 counts. They should then repeat the exercise with the opposite leg.

▌ Relevé: Exercisers begin in neutral position and rise up onto their toes (Counts 1, 2), hold (3, 4, 5, 6), bend the knees (7, 8), and hold (1, 2, 3, 4), bring the heels down flat on the pool floor (5, 6), then straighten the legs (7, 8).

▌ Balance Transfer: Standing with the feet pointing straight forward and approximately 18 to 24 inches apart, participants rise onto the toes (Counts 1, 2), transfer all the weight to the right foot (3, 4), flex the left knee and lift the left heel toward the buttocks (5, 6, 7, 8); then they hold the balance (1, 2, 3, 4), return the left foot to the pool floor (5, 6), and return to beginning position (7, 8). They then repeat the movement by transferring the weight to the left foot and lifting the right heel.

Warm-Ups at the Wall

Senior water exercisers can do warm-ups with their right or left sides to the wall, facing the wall, with their backs to the wall, or hanging onto the wall with the feet off the pool floor (neutral feet-on position. Hanging from the wall can place undue stress on shoulder joints that may already be compromised by weakness or dysfunction, so use wall-supported warm-ups where feet are off the pool floor (see Photo 5.38, p. 86) *sparingly* and always with other warm-ups between wall-supported movements. This helps to protect your seniors' shoulder joints.

▌ Side Leg Lifts: Exercisers stand, left sides to the wall, feet parallel, and lift the right leg directly to the side with some force (this creates more water resistance); then they gently lower the leg back to neutral, repeating the entire movement 8 to 10 times. Then they switch to the opposite side.

▌ Side Leg Closes: Participants do the side leg lift *except* they allow their legs to gently float open to the side and then apply force to close them back to neutral. They repeat the

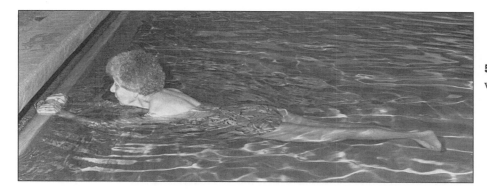

5.1a Flutter kicks facing wall.

5.1b Back to wall with legs at 90°.

5.1c Back to wall with legs out.

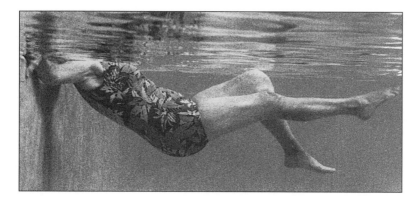

movement 8 to 10 times and then switch to the opposite side.

■ **Sunrise, Sunset:** Standing with left sides to the wall, exercisers lift the right knee to the right elbow, bending slightly at the waist to the right (Counts 1, 2), then return the right foot to the floor while extending the right arm over the head and bending slightly at the waist to the left (3, 4); they repeat the movement 8 to 10 times, and then switch to the opposite side.

■ **Flutter Kicks:** Participants face the wall with the body floating on the surface of the water and do flutter kicks (see Photo 5.1a). Vary the size and tempo of the movement from small and fast to large and slow. Kick a maximum of 1 minute at a time. This exercise can also be done with backs to the wall and arms in the pool gutter; participants flex at the hips until their legs are at a 90-degree angle (backs remain against the wall; see Photo 5.1b). An easier variation is to allow the body to come away from the

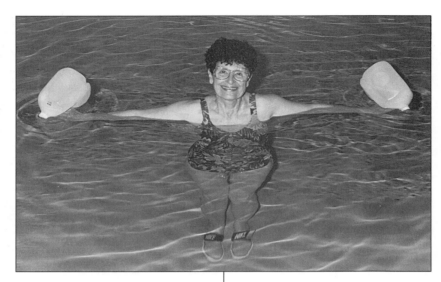

5.2   Jug work position-extended.

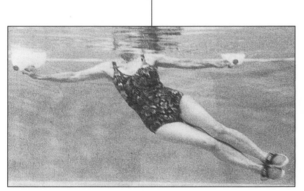

5.3   Mermaid side to side.

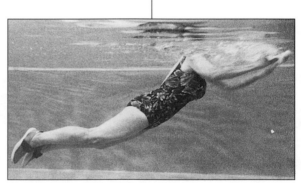

5.4   Mermaid front to back.

wall and float on the surface of the water while doing the flutter kicks (see Photo 5.1c).

JUG EXERCISES

Jug exercises are generally done in water deep enough to allow the legs to move freely without touching the bottom of the pool. Empty gallon milk jugs work very well as flotation aids. They are not to be regarded as life-saving devices, however, so those without swimming skills should not be encouraged to go to the deep end of the pool for the jug work.

Be sure to alternate jug work that requires arms to be extended at shoulder level (Photo 5.2) with those where the jug is tucked under the arm (see Photo 5.5, page 75). Keeping the

arms extended for the entire period of jug work poses unnecessary stress on the shoulder joints. Bicycling forward or backward with jugs tucked under the arms can be used between the exercises requiring arm extension. The neutral position is defined as having both legs hanging straight down. Most jug exercises can be performed for 16 to 24 repetitions.

❚ **Mermaid Side to Side:** With arms extended to the sides and legs in neutral position, the exerciser brings the knees in to the chest, then pushes both legs straight out to the right; brings knees to chest, then pushes both legs straight out to the left. The abdominal muscles are to be contracted each time the knees are brought to the chest. See Photo 5.3.

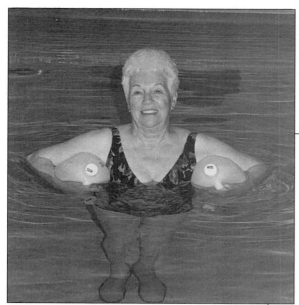

5.5 Jug work position—tucked.

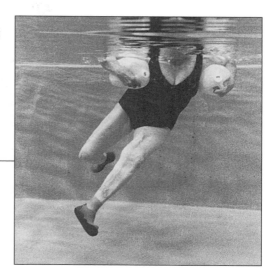

5.6 Pinwheel.

▌ *Mermaid Front to Back:* Like mermaid side to side, except legs are extended to the front and then to the back after the knees are brought to the chest. See Photo 5.4. You can offer variation by having exercisers perform a mermaid front, side, back, and side.

▌ *Pinwheel:* With the body at about a 45-degree angle and jugs either tucked under the arms (Photo 5.5) or extended to the side, the exerciser bicycles forward in a tight circle to the left, then reverses the pinwheel by bicycling backward, then switches to the opposite side and repeats. See Photo 5.6.

▌ *Bell:* With jugs tucked under the arms or extended to the sides and legs in neutral position, the exerciser pulls the knees up and out to the sides, placing the soles of the feet together. Vary the exercise by having the exerciser swing the bent legs from side to side like the ringer in a bell. See Photo 5.7.

▌ *Scissors:* With jugs tucked under the arms or extended to the sides and legs in neutral position, the exerciser opens the straight legs as far as possible (with the right going front and the left going back), then switches so the left goes front and the right goes back. You can introduce a variation using the arms in opposition to the legs. See Photo 5.8.

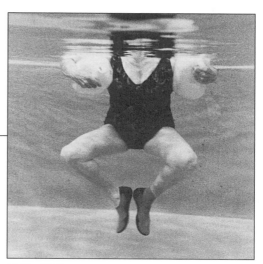

5.7 Bell.

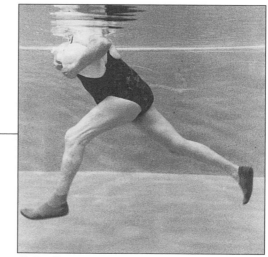

5.8 Scissors.

■ **_Pumps:_**   Beginning in neutral position with jugs extended to the sides (see Photo 5.9), the exerciser pulls the knees to the chest, extends the legs out to the front (in a sitting position), flutter-kicks the legs to an open position, and pumps the legs—right, left, right, left—by alternately flexing and extending the knees; then flutter-kicks back to a sitting position, pulls the knees to the chest, and returns legs to neutral. See Photo 5.10.

■ **_Sitting Scissors:_**   Beginning in neutral position with jugs extended to the sides (see Photo 5.9), the exerciser does the motion sequence described in the pumps but, instead of pumping with the legs while in the open sitting position, pulls the legs closed, open, closed, open; then flutter-kicks back to the sitting position, and returns legs to neutral. See Photo 5.11.

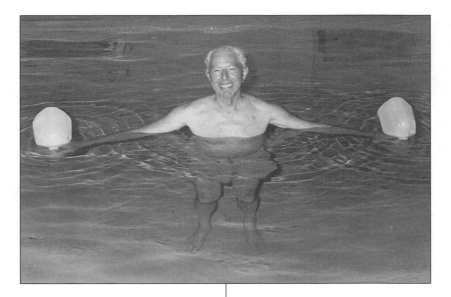

5.9   Jug work position—extended.

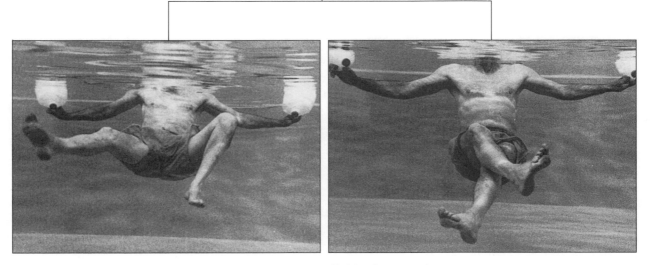

5.10   Pumps.

5.11   Sitting scissors.

■ *Open and Close Side:* With jugs extended to the sides and legs in neutral position, the exerciser opens the straight legs as far as possible to the sides, then pulls the legs closed. You can vary this exercise by using force on the open, on the close, or on both open and close.

■ *Abdominal Contraction:* Beginning in neutral position with jugs extended to the sides, the exerciser pulls the knees to the chest while contracting the abdominal muscles, then returns to neutral. Remind exercisers not to push off the pool floor with their feet.

■ *Hip Tuck:* Beginning in neutral, arms extended, the exerciser brings the knees to the chest, extends legs straight forward until lying on her back in the water, does a hip tuck by contracting the lower abdominals and tilting the pelvis under, holds the tuck 4-8 counts, then releases.

■ *Arm Jug Work:* Arm jug work is done in the shallow end of the pool in water approximately chest-deep. Keeping the jugs on the surface of the water, they can be pushed forward, then pulled back to the chest, pushed out to the sides, or pushed front and opened to the sides. You can increase the resistance by having exercisers push the jugs slightly below the water surface while performing the exercises. The jugs (either together or one at a time) can also be pushed under the water straight down toward the feet. Alternate exercises that keep the jugs on the surface with those that push them underwater. Seniors may do a maximum of 5 repetitions of pushing the jugs completely under the water. Emphasize arm jug work that takes the arms from a front extended position to one where elbows flex and pull toward the back. These contract the upper back muscles that are so important for maintaining upright posture.

AEROBICS

I have divided the aerobic exercises into four groups: the transition group (low-intensity, low-impact); Group 1 (low- to medium-intensity, low-impact); Group 2 (medium- to high-intensity, low-impact); and Group 3 (high-intensity, high-impact). To provide another measure of safety to the aerobic phase, carefully alternate transition exercises with medium- and high-intensity exercises. By structuring your class this way, you give participants an opportunity to fit the intensity of the workout to their own needs.

Transition movements can be done with minimal effort by those who wish to bring their heart rates down or more vigorously by those who wish to maintain a higher level. Frequent use of transition movements also prevents overexposure to the higher intensity "jumping" movements. Even in the water, these high-impact Group 3 exercises, when used too frequently or too long, can cause problems for those with joint dysfunction.

Transition Exercises

The transition exercise group consists of jogging in place and sculling side to side. Use these exercises to ease participants into the aerobics and then throughout the session to moderate the intensity of the workout.

■ *Jogging in Place:* Exercisers do small jogs while keeping the arm work below shoulder level. Participants who want to keep their heart rates higher can jog more vigorously, lifting their knees higher and working harder with their arms.

■ *Sculling Side to Side:* Participants do small kicks (approximately 6 inches wide) to diagonal right, left, right, left, while swaying both arms from side to side in unison with the legs. Participants who want to keep their heart rates high can kick higher and *pull* their arms through the water.

Group 1 Exercises

Group 1 exercises are low- to medium-intensity, low-impact movements. They are good exercises for beginning the aerobics phase and to use alternately with Group 2 exercises later in the session.

■ *Pendulum:* Begin with both arms to the right and parallel to the floor. Pull arms through the water like a pendulum moving to the left parallel position. Exercisers can perform this movement standing or can step from side to side in unison with arm motion (see Photo 5.12).

■ ***Rocking Horse Front:*** Exercisers rock forward on the right foot, backward on the left, using their arms (to the sides with elbows slightly flexed) to pull backward on the rock forward and forward on the rock backward; then they switch sides, rocking forward on the left foot and backward on the right. See Photo 5.13.

■ ***Rocking Horse Side:*** Exercisers rock broadly to the right side on the right foot (right arm reaching to the right), then to the left side on the left foot (left arm reaching to the left). See Photo 5.14.

■ ***Jogging Through the Water:*** Participants jog forward or backward through the water, using the resistance of the water to increase the exercise intensity.

■ ***Bicycling:*** Bicycling with jugs can be done at low intensity for the warm-up (bicycling slowly) and at higher intensity for the aerobic phase (bicycling more vigorously).

Group 2 Exercises

Group 2 exercises are medium- to high-intensity exercises with low-impact movements, which effectively elevate the heart rate without

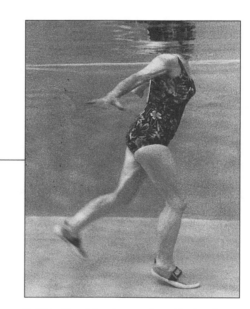

5.13 Rocking horse front to back.

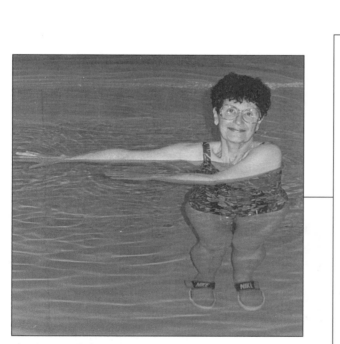

5.12 Pendulum position.

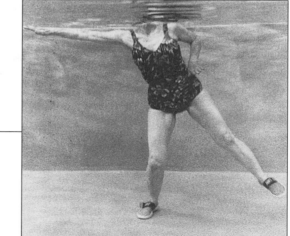

5.14 Rocking horse side to side.

any unnecessary jarring motions. Each of these exercises can be performed keeping one foot in contact with the pool floor (no jarring) or jumping from foot to foot (higher intensity with a small amount of jarring).

▌ *Knee Lifts:* Exercisers do knee lifts to the front with arms front (see Photo 5.15); or knee lifts to the sides, right elbow touching the right knee, then left elbow touching the left knee; or crossing knee lifts, left elbow touching the right knee, then right elbow touching the

left knee. See Photo 5.16 a and b.

▌ *Karate Kicks:* These are large kicks in which the right leg kicks out to the right side, then the left leg kicks to the left side. See Photo 5.17.

▌ *Front Kicks:* Exercisers do large kicks to the front with the arms pushing forward in opposition. Vary this exercise by having students reach for their shins or their toes on each kick.

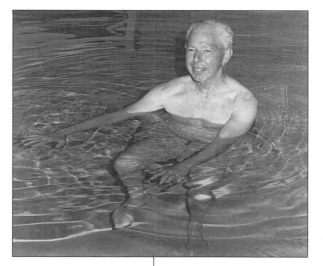

5.15 Knee lift front.

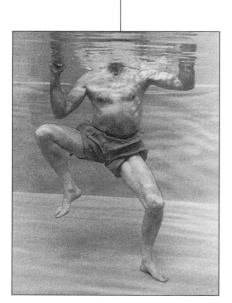

5.16a Side knee lift.

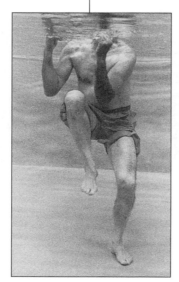

5.16b Crossing knee lift.

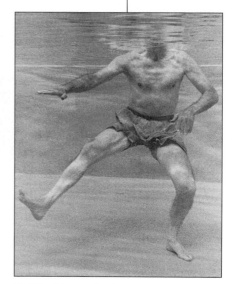

5.17 Karate kicks.

■ *Flutter Kicks:* Using the jugs, exercisers flex at the hips and do flutter kicks to the front, or with the body straight, legs outstretched behind, flutter-kick across the pool. Participants also may do flutter kicks with their back to the wall, arms in the pool gutter, or facing the wall and holding onto the pool gutter. For variety, alternate large, slow flutter kicks with small, fast flutter kicks. This exercise is most easily used at the beginning or end of the aerobic phase.

■ *Flappers Front:* See Photo 5.18 for upper body position in all flapper movements. Exercisers lift the right foot to the front and touch it with the left hand (knee is turned out to the side), and return to neutral; lift the left foot to the front and touch it with the right hand, and return to neutral. See Photo 5.19.

■ *Flappers Side:* Exercisers lift the right foot to the right side, touch it with the right hand (knee is turned in toward the center), and return to neutral; then lift the left foot to the left side, touch it with the left hand, and return to neutral. See Photo 5.20.

■ *Flappers Back:* Exercisers lift the right foot back, crossing behind the left leg, touch it with the left hand, and return to neutral; then lift the left foot back, crossing behind the right leg, touch it with the right hand, and return to neutral. See Photo 5.21.

Group 3 Exercises

Group 3 includes high-intensity, high-impact movements. The term *high-impact* is used comparatively rather than literally, because the water prevents *all* movements from being truly high impact. Always use a transition exercise immediately before and after a Group 3 exercise. Of course, as the instructor teaching from the deck

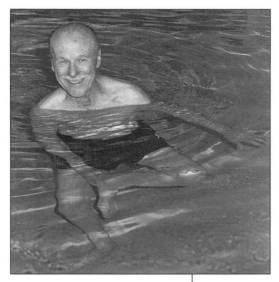

5.18 Upper body position—flappers.

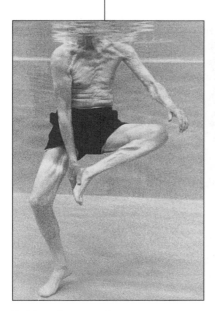

5.19 Flappers front.

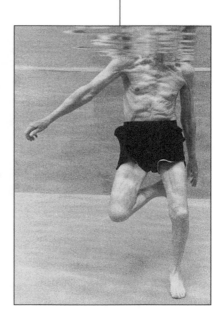

5.20 Flappers side.

5.21 Flappers back.

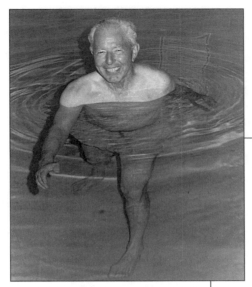

5.22 Cross-country skier—upper body.

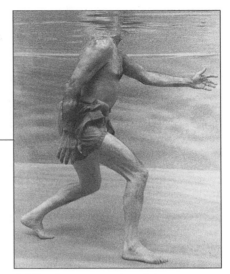

5.23 Cross-country skier.

of the pool, you should *not* perform the high-impact exercises. Instead, demonstrate one or two of the exercises so participants are clear on what they are to be doing, and then do a low-impact version while on the deck.

▋ *Cross-Country Skier:* Exercisers alternate jumping into a lunge position (right leg forward and left leg back, then left leg forward and right leg back) while swinging the arms in opposition. See Photo 5.22 for upper body position and Photo 5.23 for a side view of underwater position.

▋ *Cross Jump:* Exercisers jump up and land with the feet crossed and the arms crossed in front, then jump up and land with the feet and the arms open to the sides. See Photo 5.24.

▋ *Frog Jump:* Exercisers pull both feet up under the body at the same time with the knees pointing out to the sides, then return to a standing position. See Photo 5.25.

▋ *Jumping Jack:* Exercisers perform a standard jumping jack, arms opening to the sides as the legs open and closing next to the body as the legs come together. They can also open the arms to the sides on the jump open and cross them in front on the jump together.

▋ *Tuck Jump:* Exercisers pull both feet up together while bringing the knees to the chest into a tuck position, arms wrapped around the knees; then recover to a standing position.

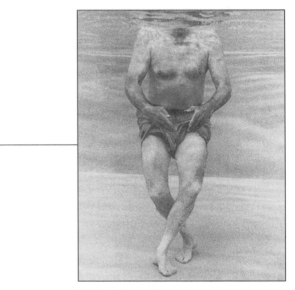

5.24 Cross jump.

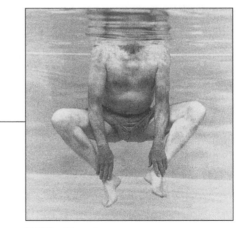

5.25 Frog jump.

▌ *Jump:* With feet together, exercisers make small jumps forward and backward or side to side.

▌ *Double Knee Bounce:* Exercisers lift the right knee while hopping on the left foot, then jump with feet together, do another right knee lift while hopping on the left foot, then jump with feet together. Repeat the movement lifting the left knee.

▌ *Traveling Movements:* Exercisers may also do jumping jacks, frog jumps, and tuck jumps while moving through the water, which makes them even higher-intensity exercises because of the increased resistance. However, use traveling Group 3 exercises very sparingly.

Cool-Down

The cool-down phase consists of slow, controlled movements that bring the heart rate down slowly and stretching exercises that help maintain or increase range of motion. Stretching exercises can be performed both in the center of the pool and at the pool wall. Relaxation movements are an excellent way to finish the class.

Center Pool

▌ *Water-Walking:* Exercisers walk slowly back and forth across the pool until the heart rate drops 4 to 5 beats below the exercise heart rate. Water-walking works very well as a transition between the aerobic phase and the cool-down and before taking the recovery heart rate.

▌ *Slow Bicycling:* Using the jugs for flotation, exercisers bicycle slowly forward and backward.

Many of the warm-up movements that focus on range of motion can also be used in the cool-down phase (e.g., the shoulder movements, arm swings, neck movements, torso contraction, balance work, and knee cross). During the cool-down phase, gently work to increase flexibility rather than just pass through a range of motion. For interest and variety, exercisers can do some of the cool-down movements while standing in a circle.

Neutral position is standing with the weight distributed evenly on both feet, arms hanging in a relaxed position to the sides.

▌ *Ear to Shoulder:* Exercisers gently drop right ear toward right shoulder, return to neutral; left ear toward left shoulder, return to neutral; chin toward the chest, return to neutral. (The shoulders must remain down in a relaxed position throughout the exercise.) Use a slow, 8- to 12-count hold in each position.

▌ *Cross Arm:* Exercisers reach the right arm across the front of the chest to the left, hold the right forearm with the left hand, and *gently* stretch the right shoulder (8 to 12 counts); then release the right arm, opening it to the right side, cross the right arm behind the back, grasp with the left hand, and hold (8 to 12 counts); release and return to neutral. They then repeat entire sequence with the left arm crossing the chest to the right.

▌ *Triceps Stretch:* Exercisers reach the right arm over the head and flex the elbow to touch the back (elbow pointing to ceiling), then reach across with the left hand and assist the triceps stretch by *gently* pulling the right elbow toward the left; they then release the arm, return to neutral, and repeat the movement on the opposite side.

▌ *Contraction:* Exercisers round the back and press grasped hands forward while bending the knees (Do *not* allow participants to sink down to round the back.) Then they straighten the back while straightening the legs and opening the arms out to sides, and return to neutral.

▌ *Balance Activities:* Exercisers rise onto the toes, balance, transfer the weight from both feet to one foot only, balance, return to both feet, then press heels down and bend the knees. To make the balance more difficult, add arm movements out to the sides and over the head.

▌ *Hug and Stretch:* Exercisers wrap the arms across the front of the chest (hug) and drop the chin toward the chest, then lift the chin to neutral while lifting the elbows up over the head and straightening the arms as if pulling a sweater off over the head, and return the arms to neutral.

▌ *Deep Breathing:* Exercisers take a deep breath in and rise up onto the toes, opening the arms to the sides; then exhale while pressing the heels back to the floor and bending the knees, one arm crossing in front and the other in back.

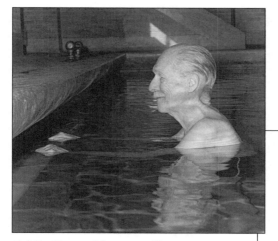

5.26 Neutral facing wall position.

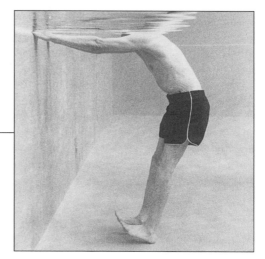

5.27 Rock backs.

▮ *Hand and Finger Mobility:* Hand and finger exercises can also be done in the water. For example, exercisers can alternately close the hand to a fist (as if grasping the water) and open the hand (as if throwing the water), do finger circles in the water (one finger at a time), pull open hands through the water, or form a circle with finger and thumb and flick the water. See chapter 4 for other wrist, hand, and finger exercises.

Wall Exercises

The positions used in wall exercises include neutral facing, neutral back, right-side neutral, left-side neutral, and neutral feet-on.

▮ *Rock Back:* Beginning in neutral facing position with hands (see Photo 5.26) gripping the gutter, exercisers rock back on the heels while flexing the feet, hold, return to neutral, then bring the chest to the pool wall while keeping the feet flat on the floor. See Photo 5.27.

▮ *Achilles Stretch:* Standing in neutral facing position, exercisers bend the right knee and place the right foot forward, simultaneously extending the left toe straight behind the body until legs are about 12 to 16 inches apart; press the left heel toward the floor, keeping the left leg straight (participants are now in a lunging position), hold for 8 to 12 counts, then return to neutral. Repeat stretch for the right leg. See Photo 5.28.

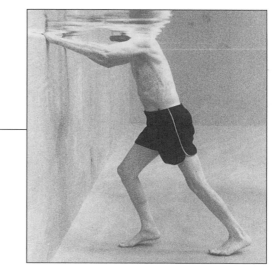

5.28 Achilles stretch.

▮ *Push Back:* Beginning in neutral facing position, exercisers flex the right knee to a 90-degree angle; keeping the abdominals engaged and the lower back straight, they press the knee back 6 to 8 inches, return to 90-degree angle. Repeat 6 to 10 times, then switch to the opposite leg. See Photo 5.29.

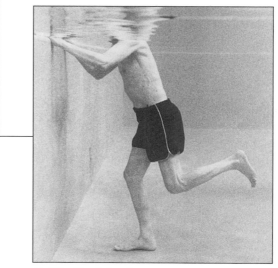

5.29 Push backs.

▌*Cross Knee:* Beginning in neutral back position (see Photo 5.30) exercisers lift the left knee to the chest (Counts 1, 2), use the right hand to bring the knee across the front of the body to the right side (3, 4), keep the shoulders square to the wall and hold (5, 6, 7, 8); then bring the knee back to center (1, 2), open to the left side (3, 4), and hold (5, 6, 7, 8); return to center (1, 2), bring the left foot back to the floor (3, 4), bend both knees (5, 6), and then straighten the knees (7, 8). They repeat the exercise on the opposite side. See Photo 5.31.

▌*Side-Lift Turnout:* Beginning in neutral back position with the right leg slightly turned out to the right, exercisers slowly lift the right leg to the right side, keeping the right heel in contact with the pool wall (this will be a small lift, if done correctly), hold, return to neutral, repeat 6 to 8 times; then they repeat the movement to the left side with the left leg slightly turned out to the left. See Photo 5.32.

▌*Hamstring Stretch:* Beginning in neutral back position, exercisers bring the right knee to the chest, then supporting the leg with the arms, extend the knee, hold, flex the foot, hold, point the toe, hold, flex the knee back to the chest, and return to neutral. Repeat the exercise without supporting the leg with the arms. Repeat the entire movement sequence with the left leg. See Photo 5.33.

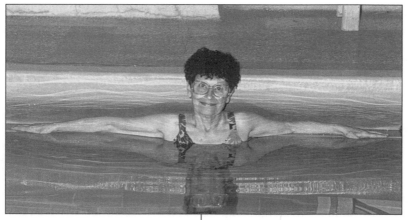

5.30 Neutral back wall position.

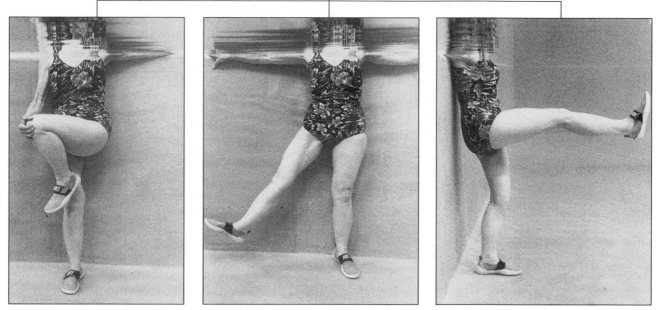

5.31 Cross kneelift.   **5.32** Side-lift turnout.   **5.33** Hamstring stretch.

■ *Hip Circles:* Beginning in neutral back position, exercisers lift the right knee up to the center, open it to the right side, and draw clockwise circles by pulling the knee back and around to the center 6 to 8 times, return to neutral, and repeat on the left side.

■ *Knee-Lift and Reach:* Standing in left-side neutral position (see Photo 5.34), exercisers lift the left knee to the left elbow, bending at the waist to the left (counts 1, 2, 3, 4), then return the left foot to the floor while extending the left arm over the head and bending at the waist toward the wall (5, 6, 7, 8); they repeat the movement slowly 4 to 6 times and then switch to the opposite side. See Photo 5.35 a and b.

■ *Quad Stretch:* Beginning in left-side neutral, exercisers bring the left heel toward the buttock by flexing the left knee. Grasp the left ankle with the left hand to hold this stretch. The left knee points straight down to the floor, and the right knee is slightly flexed. The abdominals are engaged to avoid hyperextending the back. Seniors should also avoid touching the left heel to the buttock because this hyperflexes the knee, placing it in a position vulnerable to injury. The stretch is repeated for the opposite side. See Photo 5.36.

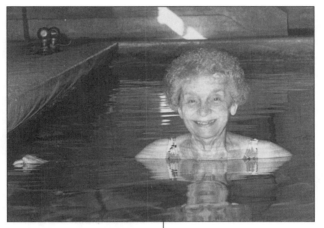

5.34 Left side neutral wall position.

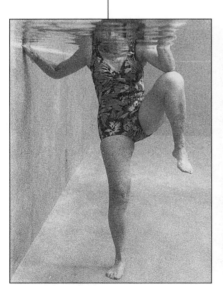

5.35a Knee lift.

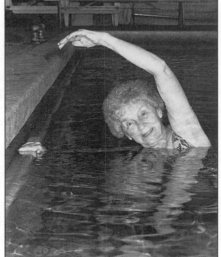

5.35b Reach.

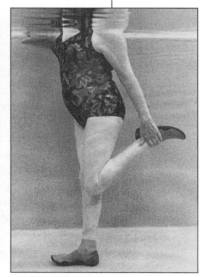

5.36 Quad stretch.

All exercises done in the left-side neutral position should be repeated in the right-side neutral position. See Photo 5.37.

Caution: *Those with back problems or shoulder abnormalities should avoid the following exercises, which require the neutral feet-on position (shown in Photo 5.38). Use these exercises sparingly with your senior population, and take care to alternate them with exercises in which the feet are on the pool floor.*

■ **Tuck Swing:**   Beginning in neutral feet-on position, exercisers gently swing the body from side to side trying to touch the surface of the water with the hip on each swing.

■ **Wall Lunge:**   Beginning in neutral feet-on position, exercisers open the legs to the side with feet far apart and, with knees pointed to the sides, lunge right, hold, lunge left, hold. The lunge-side foot should be kept flat on the pool wall to avoid hyperflexing the knee.

■ **Relaxation:**   Allow some time (3-5 minutes) for complete relaxation at the end of the class. Use relaxing instrumental music and, if possible, dim the lights. Let students float in the water, do deep breathing, or perform their choice of relaxing activities.

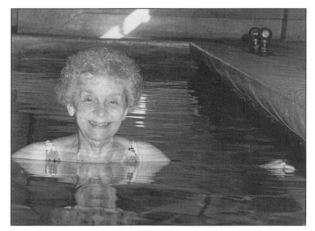

5.37   Right side neutral wall position.

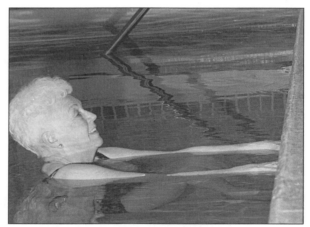

5.38   Neutral feet-on-wall position.

ARTHRITIS WATER EXERCISE

The arthritis water-exercise classes are designed to meet the needs of those who have arthritis, which significantly impairs the movement of one or more joints. These classes will also appeal to those with other physical limitations or those who prefer an exercise class that focuses on maintaining and improving range of motion and strength, aerobic conditioning being a secondary goal. Of course, because water exercise may be the only form of aerobic workout available to those with arthritis, an aerobic component should be included. The limitations in movement and the joint vulnerability posed by arthritis require special consideration be given to class format, water temperature, access needs, and specific exercise modifications.

This extra attention to detail will ensure that your program meets the special needs of this group.

CLASS FORMAT

The structure of an arthritis class is basically the same as Level 1 water exercise. It will include 20 to 25 minutes of warm-up, range-of-motion, and strength work, approximately 15 minutes of aerobics, and 20 to 25 minutes of stretching and relaxation.

The exercises described in water exercise, Levels 1 and 2, can also be used for arthritis water exercise; just keep in mind that you are dealing with individuals whose joints are significantly compromised by arthritis (see chapter 3 for information on arthritis dysfunction).

For example, arm movements must be smooth and utilize the fullest possible range of motion. Program approximately 16 to 24 repetitions of low-intensity low-impact aerobic movements and 12 to 16 repetitions of medium- to high-intensity aerobic movements with this group, and use transition movements for 16 to 24 counts between exercises. Use the high-intensity, high-impact exercises (such as jumping jacks) very sparingly, no more than 16 repetitions at a time. In addition, avoid excessive jug exercises and exercises that require students to grip the side of the pool and support their body weight with their arms and shoulders. The neutral feet-on-wall position (see Photo 5.38) should *not* be used in an arthritis class.

Finally, spend extra time asking your participants for their feedback: Is a particular exercise comfortable? Did they experience excessive soreness after the last class? (Exercise-induced soreness of the joints that lasts 2 or more hours *after* exercise is a clear indication of overexertion.) Are they achieving the results they want from class? The feedback you receive will help you help your participants gain the best results possible for the time they spend in your class.

WATER TEMPERATURE

Senior water exercise in general requires warmer than average water, and this is especially true for arthritis water exercise. Many students with arthritis become uncomfortable during the warm-up and cool-down phases of class if the water temperature is below 87 degrees. Water that is too cold can cause these students to experience discomfort and stiffness both during and after exercise. However, if the water is warmer than 90 degrees, it is too hot to include an aerobic component. Even without the aerobic component, excessively hot water (92 degrees or above) is dangerous to exercise in or even be in for long periods. Those with high blood pressure and other heart-related conditions can become dangerously overheated, which increases their risk for cardiac problems. Even those without high blood pressure can experience dizziness, nausea, and fatigue when in water that is too hot. Continually monitor the pool temperature, so you can adjust class format when necessary to ensure safety.

SPECIAL ACCESS NEEDS

A class intended for those with arthritis must be held in a pool that provides easy access. Long stairways to a pool area can be extremely difficult to maneuver for those with severe arthritis in the knees. A ladder as the only access into the pool presents an insurmountable obstacle for those with severe arthritis of the shoulders or hands. Carefully evaluate your facility to determine if you can offer a safe, accessible exercise class to this special-needs group.

JUG EXERCISES

Use of exercise jugs requires special consideration, because many class participants will have difficulty gripping and holding on to them for extended periods. Those with severe arthritis in the hands may find laundry detergent jugs and others with larger than average handles much easier to grip than the usual milk jugs. Some participants will need adult-sized water wings, foam bars, aqua bells, or some other type of flotation device instead of the jugs, due to inability to grip *any* type of jug handle.

You may need to restrict jug work to a maximum of 12 repetitions at a time to avoid excessive stress on the hands and shoulders. Also, take special care to alternate exercises that extend the arms to the sides with exercises in which the arms are bent and the jugs are tucked under the armpit. (Keeping the arms extended to the sides for too long can cause shoulder soreness.) Participants may do a maximum of two different exercises of 8 to 12 repetitions each in the extended-arm position before changing to an exercise that has the jugs tucked under the arms. Bicycling forward or backward is a good exercise to alternate with extended-arm exercises.

WALL EXERCISES

The same considerations also apply to wall work. Those with arthritis in the hands must not be expected to do wall work that requires gripping the pool gutter for long periods, so use any gutter-gripping exercises very sparingly. Avoid exercises such as tuck swings and wall lunges that require participants to be in the neutral feet-on-the-wall position (Photo 5.38). Gripping the gutter and supporting the body weight with the hands and shoulders is very difficult for those with severe arthritis in these areas. When in doubt about the appropriateness of an exercise, just weigh the benefits against the risks.

For more specific guidelines and exercises, contact the Arthritis Foundation or the YMCA to acquire their *Arthritis Foundation–YMCA Aquatic Program Instructor's Manual.* This is an excellent resource that will give you many condition-specific exercises useful to this special-needs group. Write to the YMCA Program Store, P.O. Box 5076, Champaign, IL 61825-5076, or call (800) 747-0089.

CHAPTER

6

Developing and Promoting Your Senior Exercise Program

Now that you have the programming information you need to design a safe, effective senior exercise class, you are ready to do a needs assessment and develop your program goals. Besides finding a facility that will meet the special needs of the senior population, you must devise strategies for promoting your senior exercise program and ways to motivate seniors to begin—and continue—exercising. Your careful attention to these will ensure that the time and energy you spend on developing your program is well directed.

NEEDS ASSESSMENT

Before planning a senior exercise program, take the time to assess the need in your community for such a program. Factors such as the number of seniors in your community, other programs in existence, and the demand

for exercise programming are important considerations at this stage. After you have assessed the needs of your target population, you can develop program goals that will ensure that *your* program is directed toward meeting these needs.

COMMUNITY NEEDS ASSESSMENT

First, obtain age demographics for your area from the public library, chamber of commerce, and government agencies on aging. Contact the local senior centers, recreation centers, and fitness facilities to determine what exercise programs, if any, are currently being offered to seniors. If there are senior exercise programs available, take the time to evaluate them. Call as a potential participant to see what image they project over the phone. The person who answers the telephone should be friendly and interested (but not patronizing) and project a professional image, inquiring about your current level of exercise or activity and your goals in joining the program. If possible, you should also visit the facility either as an observer or a participant. Talk to people in the program and listen to their praises and complaints. Then decide if the needs of the seniors in your community are being met sufficiently by the existing program(s).

If no program is currently available, or you determine there is a need for your program, then you must become "visible." Give talks or miniworkshops on exercise and health-related issues at the senior center, club meetings, luncheons, or special events. This also will help you determine the level of interest in a senior exercise program as well as advertise what you have to offer. And of course, you must become an integral part of the network of senior services in your community. Carefully evaluate exactly how your program will fit into the senior services network, and then establish yourself as someone serious about providing a service to seniors.

PROGRAM GOALS

Use the information you gather from your needs assessment to guide you in developing your program goals. Write down program goals and objectives, such as to increase cardiovascular fitness, strength, range of motion, balance, and coordination. Make sure that your program's efforts in these areas improve functional fitness (i.e., that level of fitness necessary to take care of personal needs, maintain independence, and engage in activities of choice). The American Alliance for Health, Physical Education, Recreation and Dance offers information on simple functional fitness testing through their Council on Aging and Adult Development. To obtain their guidelines and testing procedures write to

AAHPERD
Council on Aging and Adult Development
1900 Association Drive
Reston VA 22091

Providing a positive social experience and fostering improved self-esteem are also important objectives. Encourage your seniors toward realistic personal goals. Find out which areas of their fitness they are expecting to improve and how much they expect to improve.

Then guide your seniors toward achievable short-term and long-term accomplishments.

In addition to addressing fitness and social and emotional needs, develop program goals aimed at teaching seniors how to achieve and maintain overall wellness. Include education on nutrition, weight control, stress, and health issues specific to seniors. Be assured that the time you spend now developing your program goals will ensure a well-rounded program for your seniors.

IDENTIFYING APPROPRIATE FACILITIES

When choosing a facility for a senior exercise program, or when evaluating your own facility, you must consider its accessibility to physically restricted seniors, its appropriateness to hearing and visually impaired seniors, its capacity for proper heating and cooling, and its overall safety. A less than perfect facility should not keep you from starting a senior exercise program. It will simply mean that you need to develop your program with careful attention to the limitations of the available facility.

ACCESSIBILITY

You must evaluate your facility to determine accessibility to people with a variety of physical restrictions. The accessibility of a facility may limit who you can provide a service to. Identify any obstacles that senior clients might encounter when coming to and leaving class. Evaluate where they will park. Watch for potential problem areas, such as a long walk, difficult terrain, or stairs. Consider seasonal changes, and remember that many seniors are uneasy on snowy, slick surfaces. (Parking areas and walkways must have adequate snow removal or they become obstacles to participation.)

Scout out the route that a senior client would follow getting to and from class and determine for yourself if any of your clients would have difficulty with access. Seniors who attend low-impact aerobics class probably will not be troubled by the obstacles mentioned, but if you have a water aerobics or chair exercise program geared for those with physical limitations, you must discover and address any obstacle that might discourage or prevent their participation.

APPROPRIATENESS FOR SENIOR CLIENTS

To determine if a facility is appropriate for senior clients, you must consider the suitability of its environment for hearing and visually impaired individuals, whether the facility is in an acceptably safe location, and if the facility provides a nonthreatening environment.

A large percentage of seniors have some degree of hearing or visual deterioration; therefore you must carefully consider whether your facility minimizes or compounds these difficulties. For example, in a pool area, you will be dealing with uncorrected hearing impairments, because most seniors will not wear their hearing aids in the pool (just as those with vision difficulties probably will not wear their glasses). An environment that is noisy, due to a variety of other activities going on, can be very uncomfortable for those with hearing loss or hearing aids. Competing background noise will make it impossible to hear directions and cause increased anxiety and frustration. (Also, remember that hearing aids amplify *all* sounds, creating a jumble of noise that also will increase anxiety and frustration.) Most seniors will not return to a class that exposes them to such an uncomfortable experience. Therefore, seek out a space as free as possible from background noise and competing activities.

Seniors with poor vision or eye dysfunction are usually troubled by areas that are poorly lit or illuminated by direct sunlight or strong, reflected sunlight. Pinpoint any place in your movement area that may pose a problem, such as a surprise step-off or a sudden change in floor texture. For the visually impaired senior, an unexpected change in floor texture could mean a fall. Remember to check out parking lots and walkways when making your evaluation. Search out any surprise step-offs or level changes on the way to and from class. If classes are held at night, remember that proper lighting in the parking and walking areas is essential.

Also determine whether your environment of choice is emotionally nonintimidating and nonthreatening. For example, a facility where primarily elite athletes gather may be a poor choice for a seniors' class. Some seniors could be inspired by the exhibitions of athletic prowess, but most will likely feel inadequate and out of place. Also, scheduling a senior exercise class in an area in which they will be "on stage" (in the sense of being located where others are likely to stop and watch) can create an intimidating atmosphere, especially for beginners' classes.

In some communities, another important consideration for choosing a facility is whether it is in a safe location. A facility located in a high crime area will discourage many would-be participants.

HEATING AND COOLING

Any exercise facility must have the capacity for proper heating and cooling. This is not only an issue of comfort but also one of safety. It is dangerous for anyone to exercise in a room that is too hot. It is even more dangerous for seniors, when you consider that many have high blood pressure and other conditions that can be complicated or aggravated by the heat. Aerobic exercise done in a hot room is especially dangerous and poses an unacceptable risk to seniors. At the other extreme, a cold room makes it difficult to properly warm up the muscles, making senior participants more susceptible to muscle pulls and strains. A cold room also promotes an undesirably rapid cool-down after the aerobics and makes an uncomfortable environment for stretching and relaxation.

POOL AND SHOWER AREAS

For any water-exercise program, you must evaluate the safety and accessibility of the locker and shower areas, the pool area, and the pool itself. The locker room should be well lit, and the shower area should have a surface that minimizes slickness when wet. The pool deck should also be evaluated for slickness. A very slippery surface can pose an unacceptable risk of falling. Footwear, such as aqua shoes, often can provide better footing in areas with slippery spots, but do not allow seniors to wear old tennis shoes, which probably will have worn soles and slip on wet surfaces.

Besides the areas surrounding a pool, evaluate the access into the pool itself. A stairway should have a solid railing to assist in entering and exiting the pool. A pool that has only ladder accessibility will make climbing in and out very difficult for those with upper body limitations.

EXERCISE SURFACE

The exercise surface is of utmost importance. A poor surface can contribute significantly to gradual deterioration of the joints and the possibility of acute injury. The best surface, of course, is a suspended wood floor like that in a gymnasium or dance studio. However, in the absence of such a facility, being aware of the potential risks can help you to match the type of exercise you provide to the type of surface available.

The hardness of the exercise surface is a very important safety aspect. It is fairly common knowledge that to perform aerobic exercise on very hard surfaces, such as concrete, is unsafe. The poured floors common in some multipurpose facilities and the thin exercise matting used on such floors can also be too unforgiving on the tender knees, hips, and backs of seniors. Also, be suspicious of carpeted floors, which are often only carpet over concrete. Even the low-impact movements of a senior aerobics class should not be performed on concrete or any other hard surface that compromises already vulnerable muscles and joints.

The texture of the surface is also important. If it is slick, sticky, or has numerous slick and sticky spots, it will increase your senior exercisers' risk of falling. Carpeting also poses some challenges to safety (even when laid over an acceptable surface) requiring you to adjust your movement combinations and patterns. Movement patterns will have to be very simple

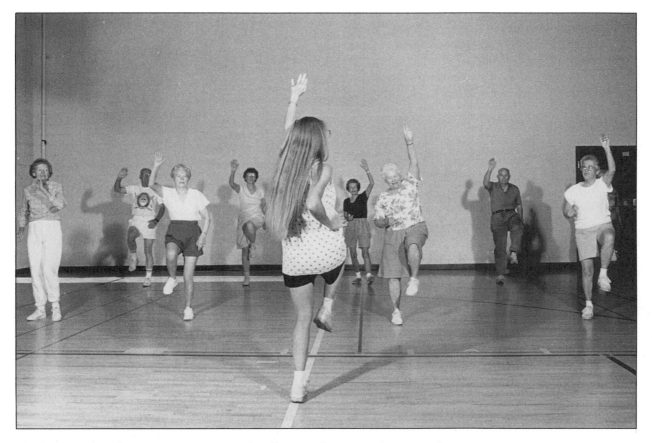

The best surface for exercising is a wooden floor such as in a dance studio or gym.

with minimal use of direction changes. Side-to-side movements, or any movement in which the foot drags across the floor, will pose a hazard. Such movements make it easy for a shoe to stick to or catch on the carpet, which can cause an ankle turn, trip, or fall. Remember: Always weigh the benefits against the risks of each movement.

LOCATING A FACILITY

If you are not already established at a particular facility, then, keeping the criteria in mind, explore local schools, churches, YMCA and YWCAs, recreation centers, colleges or universities, senior centers, and fitness clubs. You may not find the perfect facility, but when making concessions, always remember—safety first: A program cannot continue if injuries are prevalent.

You may need to modify your program to fit your facility, for example, by using energetic chair aerobics rather than low-impact aerobics, when the only exercise space available has an unsafe surface. When searching for the right movement space, do not disregard the option of providing a program without having a "base" facility. You may find it beneficial to take your program to the clients by scheduling sessions at several different places, such as senior centers, recreation centers, or senior housing facilities. You can develop a very successful program, providing exercise classes on a regular basis at a variety of facilities.

PROMOTING YOUR EXERCISE PROGRAM

Magazines and journals devoted to marketing are filled with information on how business is developing strategies for responding to the expanding older adult market. Some public relations firms are exploring the older adult market through several market segments. Consumers in their 40s, who will reach age 50 during the next decade, are considered to be on the fringe of the mature market but are still significant, because they enjoy the greatest concentration of wealth among any market segment. The 50-plus market is divided into subsegments of 50- to 64-year-olds, 65- to 74-year-olds, 75- to 84-year-olds, and, the fastest growing segment of all, the 85-plus category (Thompson, 1990). To develop the most effective public relations campaign possible, each subsegment is attributed with identifiable characteristics.

Using a different approach, Ostroff (1989) recommends that business explore the mature market's seven promising niches of need: the home, health care, leisure time, personal and business counsel, educational services, financial products and services, and products that counter aging. When planning strategies for marketing your exercise program, an "age-countering product," keep a watchful eye on how the general business world is approaching and responding to senior consumers.

DEVELOPING A NETWORK

Marketing your program will rely largely on developing a cooperative relationship with other individuals and organizations that daily provide a variety of services to seniors. One of the most beneficial steps you can take is to become an integral part of the senior services network in your community. This includes the senior center, area agencies on aging, county offices on aging, and a wide range of senior support services. If you are a visible and recognizable asset within this network, then your program will gain the credibility it deserves.

Make area physicians, physical therapists, orthopedic specialists, and chiropractors an important part of *your* network. Seek out their expertise and invite them to review your program. Ask their input on such things as the level of aerobic conditioning appropriate to seniors with heart- and lung-related restrictions, and on the safety of your exercises for particular muscle and joint conditions. Most health professionals have very time-restricted schedules, so an effective method of opening the lines of communication may be to send a letter asking a specific question that can be answered briefly. You may find a health professional who has a special interest in older adult exercise and is willing to give a little more time to answering your questions and concerns.

Strive to establish a relationship of trust and reliability. This will take time and careful attention, but it will give a great deal in return.

Adequately involving area health professionals will improve your program's safety and credibility. It may also increase participation through direct referrals from these health professionals. It is no secret that the right kind of exercise can improve many aspects of health; therefore, if area health professionals know you have a safe, effective program, they will gladly refer patients to your classes. For example, of the close to 200 participants currently involved in the Bozeman, Montana, "Young at Heart" program, approximately 40% were referred to the program by health-care professionals.

If you are fortunate enough to live close to a college or university, then include its health and fitness professionals in your network. They often can provide important up-to-the-minute information concerning specific exercise and other health-related topics and are generally more accessible than physicians. Health and fitness professionals connected with colleges and universities may also offer opportunities for participation in research projects geared toward senior exercise.

FINDING CLIENTS

To develop a marketing strategy for your program, you must decide where to focus your marketing efforts. Consider where senior consumers do business, have their health needs met, and congregate socially in your community. Once you have identified where senior consumers gather, then you can develop a marketing plan that will get your message to them.

Watch for businesses that cater to seniors with special senior discounts or extra service. Look for clothing and shoe stores, gift shops, bookstores, novelty shops, and barbers or hair designers that seniors are likely to patronize. Search out businesses that take special care to be friendly and accommodating to seniors. Some restaurants cater to older adults with special senior nights, offering additional discounts or special menus. Older cafes may be long-time favorites of seniors.

Another significant factor in why seniors patronize a business may be its location. Look for a grocery store within walking distance of senior housing or one that offers a delivery service. Also locate shopping complexes that offer one-stop shopping. Many seniors without personal transportation will frequent stores at which they can be dropped off and then take care of all of their needs in that one place.

In addition to the usual businesses, consider where the seniors in your community are likely to go for health care. Seniors consume a high percentage of prescription drugs, so find out which drugstores cater to seniors. Look for one with a convenient location or one that offers delivery service. If possible, also identify the doctors who have a large elderly clientele. These will include internists, family practice doctors, those who specialize in arthritis, and doctors that have been in the community for many years. Most doctors' offices have a bulletin board where public notices can be posted. If you have a good relationship with area physicians, many will go a step further and place posters in examining rooms or hand out your materials to those to whom they recommend exercise.

Finally, determine where the seniors in your community socialize. Senior centers, social clubs, city recreation centers, golf courses, bingo parlors, bowling alleys, special community events, and night clubs with social dance music are likely choices. Many seniors also socialize through volunteer work. Identify those community organizations whose specific focus is volunteer work, as well as organizations such as museums, hospitals, and churches. When you find out where seniors go to enjoy themselves, you will have located another place to focus your marketing efforts.

USING MEDIA TO REACH CLIENTS

After locating the seniors in your community, you are ready to develop strategies for reaching them with your program message. Newspapers, radio, and television can help you reach the senior consumer.

Because older Americans are demanding more information that is relevant to their lives, media are working hard to respond to that demand. Older adults are the most loyal readers of newspapers, and newspapers are responding by significantly increasing their coverage of aging issues. Older television viewers' preference for news, sports, talk shows, and classic movies has begun to change the programming focus of cable television from entertainment only to a mix of entertainment, news, and life-style programming. The radio industry is also taking note that

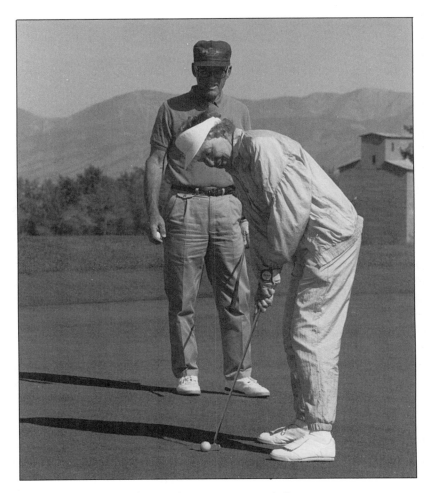

Look for clients at places where seniors socialize.

older listeners are significantly more likely to listen to all-news stations, news and talk formats, easy-listening programs, and nostalgia programs (Cutler, 1989).

Look for ways to use this relatively new media focus to promote your program. Develop a mutually beneficial relationship with the local media—the key phrase here is *mutually beneficial*—by making yourself available to them and providing background information and assistance in your area of expertise whenever asked. Then, when ready to promote your program, you can use the ongoing media interest in issues on aging to solicit local newspaper, television, and radio coverage.

Newspaper

Keep a watchful eye on any national stories concerning research on the benefits of exercise for older adults. When the national news is focusing on these types of stories, contact your local papers to see if they will run a story concerning this fitness research. Then place an advertisement about your senior exercise program to coincide with the article. If you have a program already established, this is the time to interest a local reporter in doing a feature on it as a follow-up or support article. Of course, *always* inform your local newspaper of any special events your program is planning and suggest the opportunity of a human-interest story whenever it is convenient for them.

Television

The strategies suggested for local newspaper coverage are also appropriate for drawing local television attention. The time to interest a local station in doing a feature on your program is when there is national attention focused on the benefits of exercise for older adults. You should also keep them informed of any special

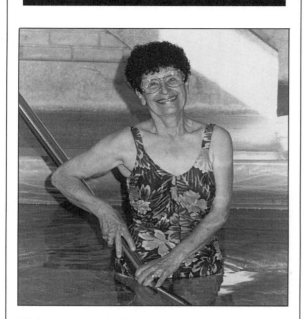

Helen, age 76, began exercising with the Young at Heart Program in Bozeman 11 years ago. She was a member of the first senior exercise class begun to research the effect of exercise on older adults. Helen takes great pride in the fact that she has been enrolled in the program every session for all of these years. Asked what motivates her to keep coming to class, she says, "The exercise classes are really a part of my life. They just make me feel so good. If I miss class I really notice a difference and can't wait until I can get back to class." She adds, "My doctor is amazed at how flexible I am, and I know it is because of the water exercise classes."

"I really enjoy the other ladies. The social aspect makes coming to class more enjoyable because I know these people and enjoy visiting with them. I also enjoy meeting the new people who come to class and am happy when they find out how much better these classes can make you feel." Helen also uses exercise equipment at home, but she wouldn't give up her water aerobics classes for anything!

events your program is planning that may suggest human-interest coverage on the local news. Area television stations may even be willing to do a live-broadcast segment, showcasing your senior exercise class in action. This can be great publicity and also a lot of fun for your senior participants.

Radio

Local radio stations can be an excellent medium for publicizing your program. Select radio stations that seniors are most likely to listen to and then plan your advertisements for when the "average senior" is likely to tune in. Many seniors get up early in the morning, and many turn on their radios. They tend to tune into news programs on a regular basis. Though radio advertising representatives will speak of "drive time" (the time that people are likely to be in their cars with their radios on), be aware that many seniors prefer to stay *off* the roads during peak traffic hours (usually 7–8 a.m., noon–1 p.m., and 5–6 p.m.). Also, many older adults avoid driving after dark. You will have to work closely with a radio advertising representative to determine the peak listening times for seniors.

Paid advertisements are not the only way to take advantage of radio. Try providing senior health tips to be read on the air during public service announcement (PSA) breaks. Simple health information followed by, "This tip is brought to you by (your local radio station) and (your program)," can do a great deal to publicize what you have to offer. Whether for an advertisement or a public service announcement, use a catchy "oldies" tune as an introduction, but make sure that the dialogue is very clearly spoken without competition from background music.

SPECIAL PROMOTIONS

Special promotions, such as connecting your program with a special community event or even a data-gathering project, can generate interest in what you are offering. They give someone who has been thinking about joining your classes a special incentive to take that first step. They can also be used to develop a core group of participants, if you are starting a new program. It is critical that you have a well-planned program in place when you pursue a special promotion, because it will initiate the beginnings of a word-of-mouth network. When this network begins, it must be overwhelmingly positive if your program is going to benefit. Any event or project used only as a publicity stunt will do more harm than good if your program cannot deliver the expected results.

One special event you can use if you have a core group of senior exercisers is to stage an exercise demonstration at the senior center or a local shopping mall. You also can hold an open house for your program, allowing potential clients an opportunity to look at your facilities and observe or try out your classes. Look for opportunities such as National Fitness Week to stage such events. Many national organizations, such as the President's Council on Physical Fitness and Sports and the American Alliance for Health, Physical Education, Recreation and Dance (AAHPERD) may have posters and other media materials you can use for such events. You can also get involved in special events sponsored by local charities or fund-raisers devoted to community projects. Often, these events are centered around a walk-a-thon or other exercise-related activity, and having your senior exercise class participate as a group can bring high visibility to your program.

It may also be beneficial to do a simple pre- and post-test data-gathering project with a group of seniors to document the effects of exercise on specific components of fitness. The AAHPERD Council on Aging and Adult Development's functional fitness test is simple and does not require specialized equipment or excessive training. Advertising for "subjects" to participate in the project can bring in new clients who have been considering joining your program and just needed an extra incentive. It also gives you the opportunity to send information updates to the local media concerning your project that can generate further interest.

On completion of the project, you will have data to use to promote your exercise program—information on improvement within the components of fitness and comments on personal progress and feelings of well-being gained through exercise. The positive results obtained by project participants will also generate a positive word-of-mouth network that can bring many new participants to your program.

PROMOTIONAL MATERIALS

You probably will use a variety of posters, flyers, and pamphlets both to help advertise your program and to communicate regularly with participants. If possible, consult a professional in marketing and graphics to help develop the best promotional materials possible. These materials will influence the first impressions your potential clients develop about the quality of your program.

Whether working with a professional or developing materials on your own, take into account the special needs of your target population. For example, a high percentage of seniors have some degree of vision loss, so you must keep the design simple, uncluttered, and easy to read. Trying to squeeze too much information onto one item will diminish the visual clarity and discourage those with vision difficulties from trying to read your brochure. Also use high contrast, such as black print on white or yellow paper; even ivory-colored paper can lessen this contrast to a significant degree. Colors such as medium to dark blue, green, and red can make print very difficult to read. Even colored inks on white paper can be difficult for seniors to read, so use black ink for the text. The print itself should be slightly larger than average and consist mostly of simple block letters. Use flowery, scripted writing sparingly, because it can decrease ease of reading. Also avoid using numerous styles of writing, which can cause a visually cluttered appearance.

Finally, have an easily identifiable logo or graphic of some sort to accompany all of your promotional materials. This gives potential clients something consistent to associate with your program and helps give it an image of permanence.

MOTIVATING OLDER ADULTS TO EXERCISE

One of the most critical components to the success of your marketing program is determining what motivates senior consumers to action. There must be motivation for them to begin your program and motivation for them to continue. Both physical and social and emotional

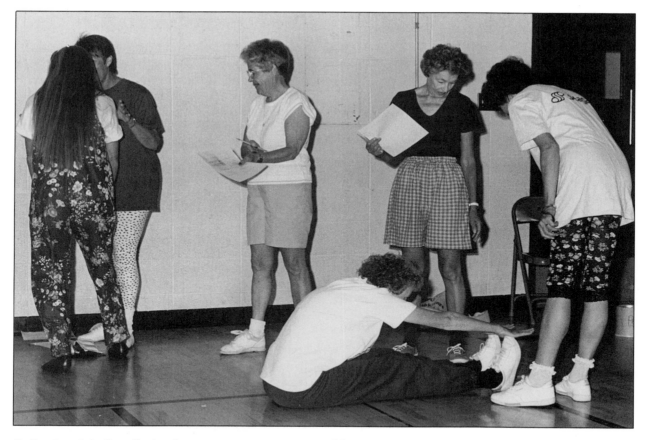

Gathering data for effects of exercise on components of fitness.

factors can motivate seniors to begin and continue an exercise program, and to achieve maximum response to your marketing efforts, you must address these aspects.

HEALTH AND PHYSICAL MOTIVATORS

Most seniors who join an exercise program are motivated by a desire to improve their functional fitness and overall health and well-being. Functional fitness involves the physical capacities necessary to maintain an independent, active life-style and positive quality of life. These capacities include range of motion, strength, balance, coordination, and cardiovascular capacity and endurance. Therefore, your program must provide "movement that matters."

You must educate seniors on how exercise benefits them specifically. For example, strength in the quadriceps muscle facilitates getting up from and down onto chairs, into and out of bed,

and walking up and down stairs with ease and confidence. Exercises that stretch the back of the calf and strengthen the front of the shin help prevent drop-foot (the slight dropping of the toe past neutral while walking), a leading cause of falls among older adults. In addition, exercises that maintain strength and flexibility in the legs can prevent gait abnormalities common in the older adult population, such as walking flat-footed or shuffling, also a leading cause of falls.

In essence, you must do your homework and know why an exercise is important and what it does specifically to improve functional fitness. Then, when advertising your program, you can emphasize how it will help seniors take an active role in maintaining and improving the physical capacities necessary to maintain their independence well into advanced age. An active, healthy, longer life is the goal—"health-span," not merely "life span."

Seniors will be motivated to continue a program if they experience noticeable improvements in physical capacities, functional fitness, or an overall feeling of improved health and well-being. If you offer a well-balanced program, they should achieve noticeable results. Solicit feedback from your group on how they feel about their progress. Determine what improvements they notice in their cardiovascular function, strength, flexibility, overall mobility, and well-being. Set up a program of minigoals for them to meet and reward their successes with prizes and minicelebrations. Give awards such as T-shirts and certificates of honor for regular attendance. Rewarding participation can provide that little extra motivation that people sometimes need to make exercise part of their healthy life-style.

SOCIAL AND EMOTIONAL MOTIVATORS

A healthy life-style involves physical well-being, mental well-being, and social and emotional well-being. Your quality seniors' program should strive to improve each of these areas. The mental well-being and social-emotional aspects of your program begin with the first phone call you receive from a senior. Project professionalism in a friendly, interested manner, giving the specific information asked for and, in turn, asking important questions about the senior. For example, ask seniors about their current level of physical condition, if they are now or have recently been involved in a regular exercise program, and what fitness goals they hope to achieve.

There are many reasons why people attend an exercise program. They may wish to improve their aerobic condition, strength, balance and coordination, or flexibility. Their goals may be less specific, like improving their overall appearance and health or improving their social life. Knowing what people hope to accomplish will help you determine how your program can best meet their needs.

When you have gathered the necessary information, explain how your program can help them accomplish their goals. If you offer a variety of classes, suggest those that will best meet their needs. This exchange of information should be conversational, not interrogative. Be prepared to visit with the client as long as necessary to obtain the needed information and to get to know a little something about this person, who may soon become part of your "family" of senior exercisers. If you answer potential clients' phone calls with impatience and or indifference, you can be sure they will *not* be motivated to take the next step—visiting your class.

When seniors come to class for the first time, ensure their warm welcome by introducing them around. You must generate a feeling of belonging among newcomers, just as you do for all participants in your program. Know your students' names and something specific about each of them, such as a special interest or talent. Make the time to visit with your students before and after classes, and take time during class for personal exchanges with and between participants. Generating a feeling of belonging to something special is the key to motivating seniors to begin and continue a senior exercise program. (See chapters 3 and 4 for specific strategies on how to address this so important component within the class format.)

References

American College of Sports Medicine. (1991a). Exercise prescription for cardiac patients. In *Guidelines for exercise testing prescription* (4th ed., pp. 121-159). Philadelphia: Lea & Febiger.

American College of Sports Medicine. (1991b). Exercise prescription for special populations. In *Guidelines for exercise testing prescription* (4th ed., pp. 161-186). Philadelphia: Lea & Febiger.

Anspaugh, D.J., Ezell, G., Rienzo, B., Varnes, J., & Walker, H. (1989). Health aspects on aging. In D.K. Leslie (Ed.), *Mature stuff: Physical activity for the older adult* (pp. 23-44). Reston, VA: American Alliance for Health, Physical Education, Recreation and Dance.

Berger, B.G. (1989). The role of physical activity in the life quality of older adults. In W.W. Spirduso & H.M. Eckert (Eds.), *The academy papers: Physical activity and aging* (pp. 42-58). Champaign, IL: Human Kinetics.

Buskirk, E.R., & Segal, S.S. (1989). The aging motor system: Skeletal muscle weakness. In W.W. Spirduso & H.M. Eckert (Eds.), *The academy papers: Physical activity and aging* (pp. 19-36). Champaign, IL: Human Kinetics.

Cutler, B. (1989, October). Mature audiences only. *American Demographics*, **11**(10), 20.

Dentzer, S. (1991, September 30). The graying of Japan: Sweeping change looms as the Asian power confronts an aging society. *U.S. News & World Report*, **8**(14), 65.

Elkowitz, E.B., & Elkowitz, D. (1986, September 1). Adding life to later years through exercise. *Exercise in the Elderly*, **80**(3), 92-94.

Goldberg, A.P., & Hagberg, J.M. (1990). Physical exercise in the elderly. In E. Schneider & J.W. Rowe (Eds.), *Handbook of the biology of aging* (3rd ed.) (pp. 407-423). San Diego: Academic Press.

Hagberg, J.M. (1988). Effect of exercise and training on older men and women with essential hypertension. In W.W. Spirduso &

H.M. Eckert (Eds.), *The academy papers: Physical activity and aging* (pp. 187-191). Champaign IL: Human Kinetics.

Kreighbaum, E. (1987). Anatomy and kinesiology. In N. Van Gelder (Ed.), *Aerobic dance-exercise instructor manual* (pp. 35-88). San Diego: International Dance-Exercise Association (IDEA) Foundation.

MacRae, P.G. (1986). The effects of physical activity on the physiological and psychological health of the older adult. In D.A. Peterson, J.E. Thornton, & J.E. Birren (Eds.), *Education and aging* (pp. 205-230). Englewood Cliffs, NJ: Prentice-Hall.

MacRae, P.G. (1989). Physical activity and the central nervous system. In W.W. Spirduso & H.M. Eckert (Eds.), *The academy papers: Physical activity and aging* (pp. 69-77). Champaign, IL: Human Kinetics.

Office of Disease Prevention and Health Promotion. (1990). *Healthy people 2000: National health promotion and disease prevention objectives*. Washington, DC: U.S. Department of Health and Human Services.

Ostroff, J. (1989, May). An aging market: How businesses can prosper. *American Demographics*, **11**(5), 26.

Pardini, A. (1987). Exercise, vitality, and aging. In H. Cox (Ed.), *Aging* (5th ed., pp. 55-65). Guilford, CT: Dushkin.

Rogers, A., Rogers, R.G., & Branch, L.G. (1989, May/June). A multistate analysis of active life expectancy. *Public Health Reports*, **104**(3), 222-226.

Rowe, J.W., & Kahn, R.L. (1987, July). Human aging: Usual and successful. *Science*, pp. 143-149.

Shephard, R.J. (1989). The aging of cardiovascular function. In W.W. Spirduso & H.M. Eckert (Eds.), *The academy papers: Physical activity and aging* (pp. 175-185). Champaign, IL: Human Kinetics.

Smith, E.L., & Gilligan, C. (1989a). Biological aging and the benefits of physical activity.

In D.K. Leslie (Ed.), *Mature stuff: Physical activity for the older adult* (pp. 45-60). Reston, VA: American Alliance for Health, Physical Education, Recreation and Dance.

Smith, E.L., & Gilligan, C. (1989b). Osteoporosis, bone mineral, and exercise. In W.W. Spirduso & H.M. Eckert (Eds.), *The academy papers: Physical activity and aging* (pp. 106-113). Champaign, IL: Human Kinetics.

Stamford, B.A. (1988). Exercise and the elderly. In K.B. Pandolf (Ed.), *Exercise and sport sciences reviews* (Vol. 16, p. 341). New York: Macmillan.

Stelmach, G.E., & Goggin, N.L. (1989). Psychomotor decline with age. In W.W. Spirduso and H.M. Eckert (Eds.), *The academy papers: Physical activity and aging* (pp. 6-18). Champaign, IL: Human Kinetics.

Thompson, F.G. (1990, February). Reaching America's aging marketplace. *Public Relations Journal,* **46**(2), 28.

U.S. Senate Special Committee on Aging. (1988). *Aging America: Trends and projections.* Washington, DC: U.S. Department of Health and Human Services.

Wells, C.L. (1987). Exercise physiology. In N. Van Gelder (Ed.), *Aerobic dance-exercise instructor manual* (pp. 3-34). San Diego: International Dance-Exercise Association (IDEA) Foundation.

Wilmore, J.H. (1988). Exercise-drug interactions in the older adult. In W.W. Spirduso & H.M. Eckert (Eds.), *The academy papers: Physical activity and aging* (pp. 194-199). Champaign, IL: Human Kinetics.

YMCA of the USA & The Arthritis Foundation (1985). Arthritis Foundation & YMCA aquatic program instructor's manual. Champaign, IL: Human Kinetics.

Index

About the Author

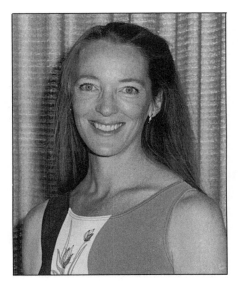

Kay Van Norman has been the director of the Young at Heart senior exercise program at Montana State University since 1988. Her responsibilities include program development and evaluation, instructor hiring and training, classroom teaching, and program promotion. She also conducts regional training workshops on the topic of senior exercise.

Kay was elected the 1995 chair of the Council on Aging and Adult Development (CAAD), a division of the American Alliance for Health, Physical Education, Recreation and Dance (AAHPERD). As the 1992 chair of the Standards Committee of CAAD, she helped to develop standards and guidelines for senior exercise instructors. Kay served as president of the Montana AHPERD for the 1991-92 term. She is also a member of AAHPERD's National Council on Aging.

Kay earned her master's degree in physical education from Montana State University in 1981. Her favorite leisure-time activities are horseback riding in the mountains, dancing, and downhill skiing. Kay, her husband, George Gebhardt, and their two children live in Bozeman, Montana.